Voice Biomarkers

Shinichi Tokuno • Hiroyuki Nakamura
Editors

Voice Biomarkers

Current Status and Issues in the Development

Springer

Editors
Shinichi Tokuno
Department of Bioengineering
University of Tokyo
Tokyo, Japan

Hiroyuki Nakamura
Ibaraki Medical Center
Tokyo Medical University
Ibaraki, Japan

ISBN 978-981-96-3108-7 ISBN 978-981-96-3109-4 (eBook)
https://doi.org/10.1007/978-981-96-3109-4

This Springer imprint is published by the registered company Springer Nature Singapore Pte Ltd.
The registered company address is: 152 Beach Road, #21-01/04 Gateway East, Singapore 189721, Singapore

Contents

Chapter 1
Overview of Voice Biomarkers

Shinichi Tokuno

1.1 Introduction

With the development and widespread use of wearable devices and smartphones, digital biomarkers that use biometric information obtained from these devices to objectively determine the presence or absence of disease and the effectiveness of treatment have been attracting attention. Voice biomarkers can be considered a type of digital biomarker and are garnering interest because voice input is extensively used, making it easier to acquire voice data. Further, significant improvement in computer technology has allowed the analysis of voice data using various devices. In addition, the COVID-19 pandemic has changed lifestyles, and living in remote environments has become more prevalent, increasing the need for such technologies (Alexa 2020). Digital biomarkers can capture information noninvasively and allow for remote intervention. In particular, voice which does not require special sensors and has a wide range of applications can be an excellent biomarker.

1.2 What Are Voice Biomarkers?

Voice refers to vibrations of air emitted from the vocal cords through the vocal tract. Humans perceive these vibrations with the help of eardrums and recognize them as voices. In digital devices, vibrations in the air are converted into electrical signals through microphones, which are then stored or transmitted as digital data to the

S. Tokuno (✉)
Department of Bioengineering, Graduate School of Engineering, The University of Tokyo, Bunkyo-ku, Tokyo, Japan
e-mail: tokuno@bioeng.t.u-tokyo.ac.jp

S. Tokuno, H. Nakamura (eds.), *Voice Biomarkers*,
https://doi.org/10.1007/978-981-96-3109-4_1

receiver. The receiver emits this digital data as voice by converting it back to vibrations of air through a speaker.

Patients with some diseases have voice modulations characteristic to the respective diseases, and voice biomarkers can be used to extract these characteristics from the analysis of voice data and help to visualize them as numerical values.

Three main types of voice are used for analysis. The three types of voices used are steady vowel sounds such as "ah~~~," voices that read out certain phrases, and voices that speak freely. The voice used for analysis was selected according to the characteristics of the disease and the purpose of voice collection.

Target diseases included otorhinolaryngological, psychiatric, geriatric, neurological, respiratory, and cardiovascular diseases. Numerous nonmedical applications have also been developed.

The voice features used in the analysis were mainly the fundamental frequency (F0) of the voice and the formant frequency, which is formed by the resonance of vocal cord vibrations as the air passes through the vocal tract. Other features that have been independently developed may also be used. A wide variety of analyses are currently being performed, and software that can analyze a large number of features are available (Eyben et al. 2010). Furthermore, by processing these features in the time direction, such as moving average, time variation (velocity), and time variation of velocity (acceleration), and by examining statistical quantities, such as mean, maximum, minimum, center of gravity, quartiles, variance, kurtosis, and skewness, a vast number of speech features can be used for analysis.

Methods used for analysis aim to search for the single most effective speech feature, for example, statistical methods such as principal component analysis and logistic regression and artificial intelligence (AI) methods such as machine learning and deep learning (Maxhuni et al. 2016).

1.3 Historical Background of Voice Biomarkers

Attempts to use voice as a biomarker have been made. In psychiatry, for example, it has been clinically noted that patients with depression have a distinctive voice quality (Newman and Mather 1938; Cobb and Lindermann 1943; Moses 1954). The first attempt to use voice as a biomarker was the spectral analysis of the voices of patients with depression by Hargreaves et al. (1965). Eventually, attempts were made to analyze the fundamental frequency (F0) of speech, and Darby et al. compared the variability of F0 between healthy individuals and patients with depression (Darby and Hollien 1977).

Tolkmitt and others compared F0 means (Tolkmitt et al. 1982). In the late 1980s, further F0 analysis was performed (Nilsonne et al. 1988; Scherer 1987). Nilsonne et al. introduced detailed methods for computer analysis of F0, and Scherer analyzed voice features such as jitter (frequency fluctuation) and shimmer (amplitude fluctuation) and found that jitter was higher in the voices of patients with depression. An analysis of the formant frequency, which is formed by the resonance of vocal fold vibrations as the air passes through the vocal tract, was conducted (Flint et al. 1993). In the twenty-first century, the harmonic-to-noise ratio (HNR), a voice feature used to assess hoarseness, has been reported to be higher in individuals with depression (Low et al. 2011).

Parkinson's disease (PD) is one of the most common diseases for which voice biomarkers are used.

Voice abnormalities in patients with PD were first described by James Parkinson in 1817, and subsequent studies have shown that patients with PD have a high rate of speech and dysarthria (Hartelius and Svensson 1994). Abnormalities in voice and dysarthria in PD are considered motor symptoms and appear relatively early in the disease (Canter 1963). The MDS-Unified Parkinson's Disease Rating Scale (UPDRS), a rating scale developed by the Movement Disorder Society (MDS), also evaluates PD using two parameters (Goetz et al. 2008). In 1963, Canter et al. reported that frequency variability was reduced when patients with PD spoke sentences. It was not until the 1990s that voice feature analysis, as we know it today, was performed, and Jiménez-Jiménez et al. reported higher jitter and shimmer and lower HNR in patients with PD (Jiménez-Jiménez et al. 1997).

In contrast, diseases that directly affect the vocal tract and cause voice disorders and dysarthria include polyps of the vocal cords, laryngeal cancer, and other otorhinolaryngological diseases. Patients with motor dysarthria or functional dysarthria of unknown cause also visited the otorhinolaryngology clinic. Therefore, the field has long used patient interviews, laryngeal imaging with stroboscopes and laryngoscopes, basic aerodynamic evaluation, perceptual analysis using standardized psychoacoustic methods, acoustic analysis, and subjective voice evaluation. Moreover, this field has also attempted to detect voice changes early using digital voice analysis. In this regard, attempts are being made to detect voice changes at an early stage through digital analysis of the voice. Clinical application of this method started in the 1970s. In Japan, the Clinical Practice Guidelines for the Diagnosis and Management of Voice Disorders 2018, which include acoustic analysis, have been published (Umeno et al. 2020).

The analysis of voice in patients with depression, PD, and dysarthria commenced in the mid-1960s, a challenging study at the time considering that personal computers were not available until the mid-1970s.

1.4 Recent Studies on Voice Biomarkers

A "voice biomarker" search in PubMed shows that 285 articles were published from June 2012 to May 2022; however, only 73 articles explicitly addressed studies on voice biomarkers. The classification of these 73 papers by disease type is presented in Table 1.1. The largest number of papers are on PD due to its historical background and ease of detection. This is followed by stress-related diseases such as depression and post-traumatic stress disorder (PTSD), cardiovascular diseases such as heart failure, and aging-related diseases such as dementia. Recently, attempts

Table 1.1 Number of papers on speech biomarkers published from June 2012 to May 2022 by domain

Category	Target diseases	Number of papers
Neurology (20)	Parkinson's disease	16
	Ataxia	2
	Multiple sclerosis	1
	Neurogenerative disease	1
Psychiatry (18)	Depression	9
	Stress	2
	Autism	2
	PTSD	1
	Bipolar disorder	1
	Manic disorder	1
	Schizophrenia	1
	Apathy	1
Cardiology (6)	Heart failure	3
	Coronary artery disease	2
	Pulmonary hypertension	1
Geriatrics (5)	Dementia	4
	Aging	1
Respiratory (5)	COVID-19	4
	Acute respiratory illness	1
Otorhinolaryngology (2)	Spasmodic dysphonia	1
	Vocal fold paralysis	1
Pediatrics (2)	Development	1
	Isolated growth hormone deficiency (IGHD)	1
Internal medicine (2)	Vitamin D deficiency	1
	Diabetes mellitus	1
Psychology (2)	Communication	1
	Trance	1
Physiology (2)	Differentiate gender	2
Gynecology (1)	Menstrual cycle	1
Occupational health (1)	Workplace environment	1
Animal experiment (1)	Ultrasonic vocalization (USV)	1

have been made to detect acute respiratory disorders in COVID-19 patients using voice biomarkers. Notably, six reviews indicated the depth of interest in this area. As shown in Table 1.2, there has been a sharp increase in the number of publications in this field since 2020, probably because the term "voice biomarker" became popular around this time.

In a recent report on stress-related disorders such as depression, which has been the focus of our research to date, Zhang used a web-based audio collection of 222

Table 1.2 Number of papers on voice biomarkers published from June 2012 to May 2022 by year of publication

Publication year	Number of papers
2014	1
2015	0
2016	2
2017	3
2018	6
2019	7
2020	21
2021	19
2022	14

individuals to create a model for predicting psychomotor disorders, suicidality, and depression severity, as indicated by the Patient Health Questionnaire (PHQ9) scores (Zhang et al. 2020). They extracted voice features using open-source Speech and Music Interpretation by Large-space Extraction (OpenSMILE) and evaluated them using multiple statistical models. Ozkanca created a model to predict symptoms of depression from voice in 921 people with PD. Sverdlov et al. assessed depression using multiple digital devices, including EEG, eye movements, and self-administered questionnaires, in addition to voice analysis (Sverdlov et al. 2021). They reported that the Sonde Health system had an area under the curve (AUC) of 0.72 on a logistic model basis and AUC = 0.69 on a linear model basis. Lee et al. assessed depression in the elderly using machine learning for voice features (Lee et al. 2021). Schultebraucks built a predictive model for PTSD symptoms using deep learning voice analysis (Schultebraucks et al. 2020). Slavich presented a general review of voice stress biomarkers and pointed out that they were not adequately comparable to blood biomarkers (Slavich et al. 2019). On the other hand, Kunin, in his general review, mentioned the possibility of automatic analysis of voice recordings via artificial intelligence (AI)-based system to derive digital biomarkers of stress from the investigation of physical changes during stress (Kunin et al. 2020).

1.5 Clinical Application of Voice Biomarkers

We have studied voice biomarkers for the detection of stress, depression, post-traumatic stress disorder, bipolar disorder, PD, dementia (including mild cognitive impairment), laryngeal deviation, sleep apnea syndrome, and COVID-19. Other applications include the prediction of driving skills in the elderly and mental healthcare for athletes. This document describes these in detail in the following chapters; however, an overview of clinical applications is provided below.

1.5.1 Stress and Depression

In 2017, we developed and released the mind monitoring system (MIMOSYS), a smartphone application that estimates symptoms of stress and depression based on the emotional components of voice, and conducted various validations (see Chap. 2). We are also developing a voice biomarker for depression that is not mediated by emotion (see Sect. 1.3). We have already developed several original voice features and are developing voice biomarkers based on more voice features using statistical methods and machine learning. Currently, these methods are being validated for practical applications.

1.5.2 Bipolar Disorder

Patients with bipolar disorder often visit a clinic during the depressive phase. However, it is often difficult to diagnose bipolar immediately because individuals are unaware that they are bipolar. It has been reported that 65% of patients with bipolar disorder had an initial diagnosis of depression (Watanabe et al. 2016). We believe that if we could suggest the possibility of bipolar disorder based on the voice at the time of initial diagnosis, it would lead to effective treatment. Therefore, we analyzed and compared the voices of patients in the depressed phase of bipolar disorder, patients with major depression, and healthy subjects. Using the prediction model obtained from the analysis, we classified the patients into three groups with an accuracy of 90.79% (see Chap. 12).

1.5.3 Post-traumatic Stress Disorder (PTSD)

There have been many studies on the use of voice biomarkers for the detection of PTSD (Low et al. 2020). In particular, many studies have been conducted in the United States on PTSD patients from the military after the Iraq and Afghanistan wars. Based on our own experience of PTSD among dentists due to their work with dead bodies after the Great East Japan Earthquake, we also assessed stress during training of dentists and other personnel for the identification of dead bodies using analysis of the voice of the individuals (see Chap. 13). Although this training was conducted using cadavers, we found that the degree of stress when in contact with cadavers varied depending on the participants' experience and order of training.

1.5.4 Parkinson's Disease

Stuttering is a major symptom of PD, and the voice of patients with PD has been analyzed for several years; even today, many studies are focusing on such voice analysis (see above). We also studied the voice of a small number of patients with PD and were able to detect PD with 95.2% accuracy using a machine learning model, with 93% sensitivity and 94% specificity with our voice features (see Chap. 14).

1.5.5 Dementia

Early detection and slowing the progression of dementia are the mainstays of dementia treatment. Therefore, we focused on the detection of mild cognitive impairment. However, while dementia can be detected by comparing voices alone, accuracy in detecting mild cognitive impairment is inadequate. We obtained adequate accuracy by imposing a computational task and comparing it to a voice without the task (see Chap. 15). A prototype of a smartphone application using this technology has been developed and is being tested for practical use.

1.5.6 Sleep Apnea Syndrome

The definitive diagnosis of sleep apnea is made using polysomnography (PSG), which requires an overnight hospital stay and is not easy to perform. A simple screening test (Apnomonitor) is also available; however, this also requires an outpatient visit. As a more convenient method, we attempted voice analysis using a smartphone. Good results were obtained by comparing voices in the sitting and supine positions (see Chap. 17).

1.5.7 Anomalous Displacement of the Tongue, Epiglottis, and Larynx (ADEL)

Anomalous displacement of the tongue, epiglottis, and larynx (ADEL) is thought to be one of the causes of abnormal crying and is also thought to be a cause of abuse. Voice before and after correction of the epiglottis and larynx (CGL) showed improvement. Laryngomalacia is the most common cause of inspiratory stridor in infancy, and analysis of crying voices showed that it could be determined with 83.8% accuracy (see Chap. 18).

1.5.8 Prediction of Driving Skills in the Elderly

We compared the driving skills, cognitive function (MMSE: Mini-Mental State Examination), and voice of 45 elderly people who drove regularly using a driving simulator. No correlation was found between cognitive function and driving skills; however, the voice index we developed could distinguish between individuals with high and low driving skills with adequate accuracy (see Chap. 20).

1.5.9 Others

Mental Care for Athletes
MIMOSYS has been used as a mental conditioning tool for archery Olympic qualifiers and female rugby players. It has been confirmed that a decline in the mental state of athletes reflects in the voice before a decline in their performance.

COVID-19
Patients infected with the novel coronavirus, nCOV-2, who have mild symptoms or are asymptomatic and are recuperating at home are followed up by confirming symptoms by telephone or other means. In such individuals, blood oxygen saturation is important, however, it is difficult to distribute pulse oximeters to all home care patients because of the large number of infected patients. Therefore, we examined whether it would be possible to determine the severity of the illness based on voice analysis.

1.5.10 Conclusion

Voice biomarkers can serve as an alternative to medical devices, which are not widely available in every household or as a means of providing objective indicators for diseases that can only be judged subjectively. If the use of voice biomarkers becomes common, it will help healthy people and patients in their self-care, and it will be possible to make users aware of their condition and help them improve their lifestyle or seek medical attention at an early stage. Furthermore, if the accuracy of this technology is improved, it could become a new decision-making tool for physicians. The development of voice biomarkers is relatively easy if the voices of patients and controls are properly labeled with the diagnosis and severity of illness. We look forward to the expansion of voice biomarker research in various medical fields.

References

Alexa EA (2020) Do I have COVID-19? Nature 2020(586):22–25
Canter GJ (1963) Speech characteristics of patients with Parkinson's disease: I. Intensity, pitch, and duration. J Speech Hear Disord 28(3):221–229
Cobb S, Lindemann E (1943) Neuropsychiatric observations. (In a symposium on the management of the Cocoanut Grove bums at the Massachusetts General Hospital). Ann Surg 117(2):814
Darby JK, Hollien H (1977) Vocal and speech patterns of depressive patients. Folia Phoniatr Logop 2(9):279–291
Eyben F, Wöllmer M, Schuller B (2010) Opensmile: the Munich versatile and fast open-source audio feature extractor. In: Proceedings of the 18th ACM international conference on multimedia. ACM, pp 1459–1462
Flint AJ, Black SE, Campbell-Taylor I, Gailey GF, Levinton C (1993) Abnormal speech articulation, psychomotor retardation, and subcortical dysfunction in major depression. J Psychiatr Res 27(3):309–319
Goetz CG, Tilley BC, Shaftman SR, Stebbins GT, Fahn S, Martinez-Martin P, LaPelle N (2008) Movement Disorder Society-sponsored revision of the Unified Parkinson's Disease Rating Scale (MDS-UPDRS): scale presentation and clinimetric testing results. Movement Disord 23(15):2129–2170
Hargreaves W, Starkweather J, Blacker K (1965) Voice quality in depression. J Abnorm Psychol 70:218–220
Hartelius L, Svensson P (1994) Speech and swallowing symptoms associated with Parkinson's disease and multiple sclerosis: a survey. Folia Phoniatr Logop 46(1):9–17
Jiménez-Jiménez FJ, Gamboa J, Nieto A, Guerrero J, Orti-Pareja M, Molina JA et al (1997) Acoustic voice analysis in untreated patients with Parkinson's disease. Parkinsonism Relat Disord 3(2):111–116
Kunin A, Sargheini N, Birkenbihl C, Moiseeva N, Fröhlich H, Golubnitschaja O (2020) Voice perturbations under the stress overload in young individuals: phenotyping and suboptimal health as predictors for cascading pathologies. EPMA J 11(4):1–11
Lee S, Suh SW, Kim T, Kim K, Lee KH, Lee JR, Han G, Hong JW, Han JW, Lee K, Kim KW (2021) Screening major depressive disorder using vocal acoustic features in the elderly by sex. J Affect Disord 1(291):15–23
Low LSA, Maddage NC, Lech M, Sheeber LB, Allen NB (2011) Detection of clinical depression in adolescents' speech during family interactions. IEEE Trans Biomed Eng 58(3):574–586
Low DM, Bentley KH, Ghosh SS (2020) Automated assessment of psychiatric disorders using speech. A systematic review. Laryngosc Investig Otolaryngol 5(1):96–116
Maxhuni A, Muñoz-Meléndez A, Osmani V, Perez H, Mayora O, Morales EF (2016) Classification of bipolar disorder episodes based on analysis of voice and motor activity of patients. Pervasive Mobile Comput 31:50–66
Moses PJ (1954) The voice of neurosis. Grune and Stratton, New York
Newman SS, Mather VG (1938) Analysis of spoken language of patients with affective disorders. Am J Psychiatry 94:912–942
Nilsonne Å, Sundberg J, Ternström S, Askenfelt A (1988) Measuring the rate of change of voice fundamental frequency in fluent speech during mental depression. J Acoust Soc Am 83(2):716–728
Scherer KR (1987) Vocal assessment of affective disorders. In: Maser JD (ed) Depression and expressive behavior. Lawrence Erlbaum Associates, pp 57–82
Schultebraucks K, Yadav V, Shalev AY, Bonanno GA, Galatzer-Levy IR (2020) Deep learning-based classification of posttraumatic stress disorder and depression following trauma utilizing visual and auditory markers of arousal and mood. Psychol Med 3:1–11
Slavich GM, Taylor S, Picard RW (2019) Stress measurement using speech: recent advancements, validation issues, and ethical and privacy considerations. Stress 22(4):408–413

Sverdlov O, Curcic J, Hannesdottir K, Gou L, De Luca V, Ambrosetti F, Zhang B, Praestgaard J, Vallejo V, Dolman A, Gomez-Mancilla B, Biliouris K, Deurinck M, Cormack F, Anderson JJ, Bott NT, Peremen Z, Issachar G, Laufer O, Joachim D, Jagesar RR, Jongs N, Kas MJ, Zhuparris A, Zuiker R, Recourt K, Zuilhof Z, Cha JH, Jacobs GE (2021) A study of novel exploratory tools, digital technologies, and central nervous system biomarkers to characterize unipolar depression. Front Psychiatry 6(12):640741

Tolkmitt F, Helfrich H, Standke R, Scherer KR (1982) Vocal indicators of psychiatric treatment effects in depressive and schizophrenics. J Commun Disord 15:209–222

Umeno H, Hyodo M, Haji T, Hara H, Imaizumi M, Ishige M, Kumada M, Makiyama K, Nishizawa N, Saito K, Shiromoto O, Suehiro A, Takahashi G, Tateya I, Tsunoda K, Shiotani A, Omori K (2020) A summary of the Clinical Practice Guideline for the Diagnosis and Management of Voice Disorders, 2018 in Japan. Auris Nasus Larynx 47(1):7–17

Watanabe K, Harada E, Inoue T et al (2016) Perceptions and impact of bipolar disorder in Japan: results of an Internet survey. Neuropsychiatr Dis Treat 12:2981

Zhang L, Duvvuri R, Chandra KKL, Nguyen T, Ghomi RH (2020) Automated voice biomarkers for depression symptoms using an online cross-sectional data collection initiative. Depress Anxiety 37(7):657–669

Chapter 2
Stress and Depressive Symptoms: Development of Psychoanalyzer

Mitsuteru Nakamura

2.1 Introduction

It is known that response personnel deployed in disaster areas are subjected to excessive stress, which can lead to mental disorders such as post-traumatic stress disorder and depression (Raphael et al. 1984; Fullerton et al. 2004; Perrin et al. 2007; Dobashi et al. 2014). A high frequency of mental health assessment is necessary to protect them from mental illness. Various methods have been proposed to assess mental status, but these methods must be noninvasive and low-cost, taking into account the burden on the subject to be assessed if they are to be conducted at high frequencies.

In addition to the spontaneous changes associated with internal activities, human emotions are also influenced by the external environment, such as excessive stress (Lazarus 1993). Although there is a great diversity in emotions, the general theory is that the influence of the external environment on emotions appears as differences between groups of people in different environments. Just as people routinely learn about the emotions of others in a noncontact manner, emotions may be measured using noncontact means that do not involve physical contact with the subject, which is much less invasive. Many biomarkers involve physical invasion or contact, and many require expensive consumables.

One method for measuring human emotion is to measure activity in areas of the brain thought to be related to emotion (Phillips et al. 1998), but this generally requires expensive equipment and is not suitable for everyday use.

Low-cost emotion measurement techniques used in daily life include facial expression recognition (Tian et al. 2011) and voice analysis (Mitsuyoshi et al. 2006,

M. Nakamura (✉)
Department of Bioengineering, Graduate School of Engineering, The University of Tokyo, Bunkyo-ku, Tokyo, Japan
e-mail: nakamura@bioeng.t.u-tokyo.ac.jp

S. Tokuno, H. Nakamura (eds.), *Voice Biomarkers*,
https://doi.org/10.1007/978-981-96-3109-4_2

2007; Mitsuyoshi 2008). Although facial expression recognition is relatively easy to recognize in the same person, it is difficult to recognize between different individuals because of individual differences, making general use without customization difficult. There is also a bias between cultures in facial expression (Elfenbein and Ambady 2002). One study that attempted to measure stress from facial expressions (Gao et al. 2014) considered anger and disgust collectively as equivalent emotions as markers of the presence of stress and did not compare them to questionnaires or other biomarkers.

Although there is diversity in the expression of emotions through speech owing to individual differences, Sensibility Technology (ST) (Mitsuyoshi et al. 2006, 2007; Mitsuyoshi 2008), a speech emotion recognition technology, overcomes individual differences by obtaining samples from a large number of people. In addition, ST does not depend on the linguistic content of speech and has a wider range of potential applications.

If speech emotion recognition with ST can achieve the same or higher accuracy than the subjective emotion ratings of the target person, we can expect to detect the emotional impact caused by mood disorders with the same or higher accuracy than subjective questionnaires.

Based on this hypothesis, we developed vocal affect display (VAD) as a speech biomarker derived from speech emotion recognition, which is an overall indicator of emotion and reflects changes due to environmental influences. The VAD was developed using three indicators: low VAD (VAD-L), which indicates overall negative mood; high VAD (VAD-H), which indicates overall positive mood; and the VAD ratio (VAD-R), which is the ratio of the three indicators. As a preliminary study to verify the applicability of the VAD, we collected voice data from Japanese Self-Defense Forces personnel who were deployed to Haiti for disaster relief following the 2010 earthquake and investigated the relationship between the VAD calculated from their voices and the length of their deployment.

2.2 Methods

ST software ver. 3.0 (AGI Inc., Tokyo, Japan) was used to analyze participants' speech and measure their emotions.

The emotion factors detected by the ST software were anger, joy, sadness, calmness, and excitement. The output of the software was the intensity of each emotion detected in the input speech, expressed as an integer value between 0 and 10. A value of 0 indicates that the input speech does not contain emotion, whereas a value of 10 indicates that the emotion in the input speech is extremely strong.

ST software was developed based on the idea that excitement differs from the other four emotions, which means that it contains an element that is also related to the other four emotions: the degree of arousal (Mitsuyoshi et al. 2006). The ST software outputs values for the four emotions, other than excitement, as a percentage of a given emotion for all four emotions. For example, if the degree of joy is reduced, the total value of the degree of the three emotions other than joy will increase accordingly. We treat the degree of excitement as the most important indicator of VAD.

The smallest unit of speech analyzed by the ST software is the "utterance," which refers to the sequence of speech utterances from one breath-hold to the next. For implementation purposes, the onset of speech is defined as a change from a state in which the volume is sufficiently low to be considered silent to a state in which the volume is sufficiently high to be considered the onset of speech, and the state continues for a certain period of time. End-of-speech is defined as a change from a state in which the volume is sufficiently high to be considered a speech state to a state in which the volume is sufficiently low to be considered silent and continues for a certain period of time after the speech is judged to have begun. In this study, the threshold values for the silence and speech states were determined on a case-by-case basis after listening to the recorded data, because the volume level varied depending on the participants and the recording conditions.

2.2.1 *Algorithms for Calculation of Vocal Affect Display Indices*

The output of the ST software is the intensity of individual emotions and not the overall emotional state. We defined three indicators to indicate the overall emotional state, which we named vocal affect display (VAD). Two of the three indicators were negative and positive emotional states: low VAD (VAD-L) and high VAD (VAD-H). The other indicator was the VAD ratio (VAD-R), created for screening purposes.

The details of the algorithm are shown in the flowchart in Fig. 2.1. The input variables are the output values from speech emotion recognition by ST. The types of emotions are abbreviated as anger, A; joyfulness, J; calmness, C; sorrow, S; and degree of excitement, E, respectively. Each value was expressed as an integer between 0 and 10. The two types of VAD outputs by the algorithms shown in Fig. 2.1 are abbreviated as low VAD (VAD-L): L and high VAD (VAD-H): H.

The first algorithm computes an index that reflects the degree of emotion strongly associated with an overall depressed (low) emotional state. The second algorithm computes an index that reflects the degree of emotion strongly associated with an overall high emotional state. Both algorithms look first at the degree of excitement (E) output by the ST and then at the overall composition of emotions by focusing on the differences in the intensity of each emotion.

These algorithms were constructed based on the fact that the degree of excitement, which the ST finds primarily using acoustic features related to the fundamental frequency, reflects the intensity of activity in the areas of the brain responsible for emotion and indicates the overall intensity of emotion. Because the main feature of the pathophysiology of mood disorders is the loss of emotional expression, we

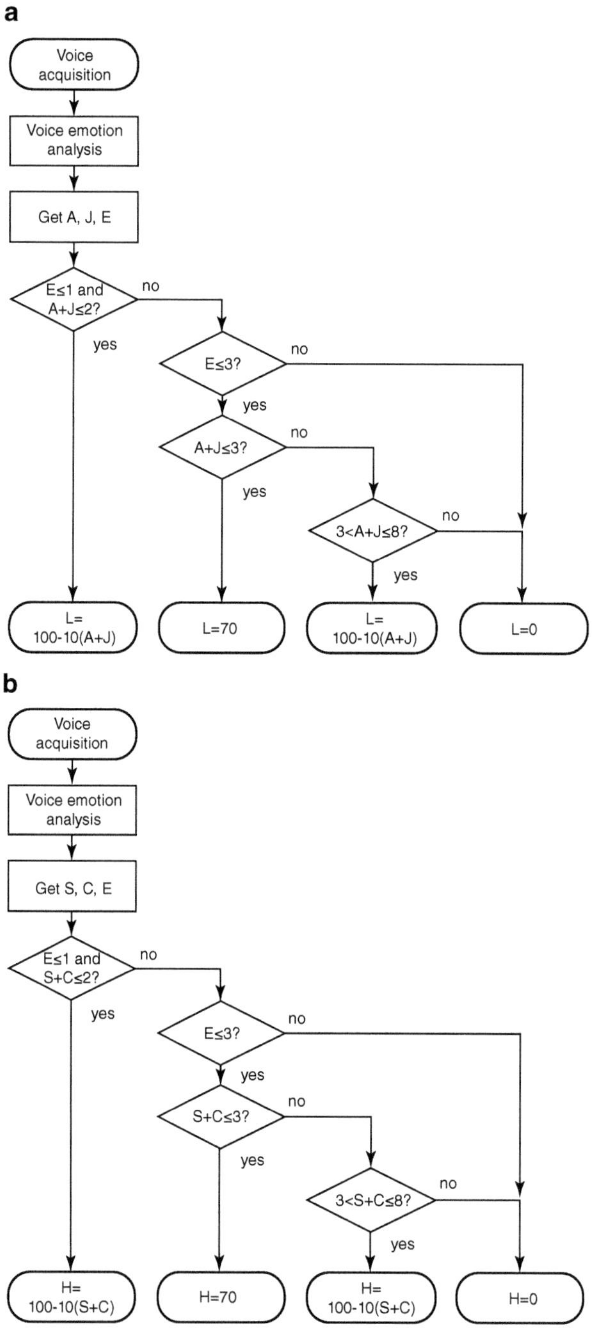

Fig. 2.1 Flowchart of the proposed algorithms. (**a**) algorithm for calculation of VAD-L; (**b**) algorithm for calculation of VAD-H. Abbreviations are as follows: VAD-L (L), VAD-H (H), anger (A), joy (J), excitement (E), sorrow (S), and calm (C). (Modified from Mitsuyoshi et al. 2017)

hypothesized that it would be useful to infer the intensity of emotion in the brain based on the degree of excitation to capture this feature.

We hypothesized that a low emotional state and emotional inactivity are present when the degree of arousal, E, is 3 or less on a 10-point scale and that emotions are extremely reduced or lost when E is one or less. Based on this process, the upper limit of E for the low emotional state was set to three, and the upper limit of E for the most severe state was set to one. These thresholds were selected based on patients' speech characteristics (such as unstable or barely audible voice and lack of vitality), which one of the authors (Mitsuyoshi et al. 2017) has observed and heard during interviews of depressed patients with clinical psychologists and physicians since 2002.

We define a session as a group of multiple utterances that are temporally continuous. We then created an interface to visualize the short-term changes in the VADs obtained from the two algorithms described above for each utterance and the long-term trend averaged over the entire session. An example of this interface is shown in Fig. 2.2.

For any given series of sessions, the ratio of the within-session average VAD-H to the within-session average VAD-L was defined as the VAD-R for that session.

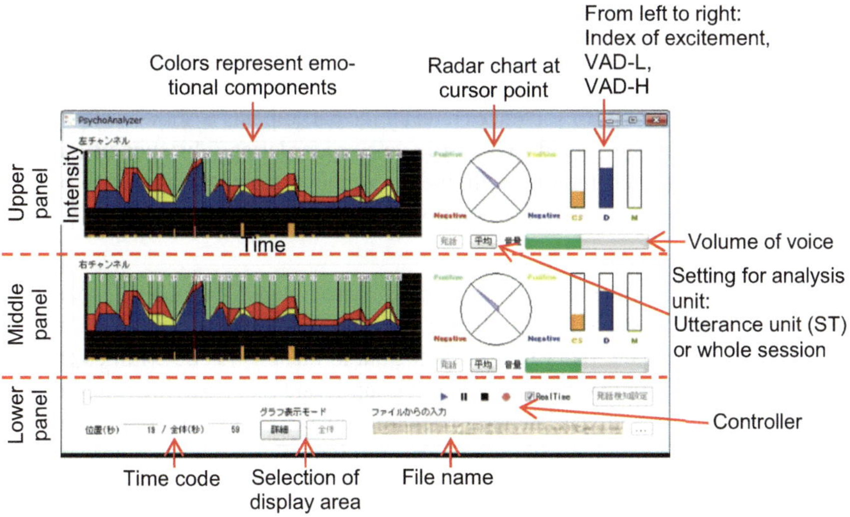

Fig 2.2 User interface of Psychoanalyzer. The application was developed for Japanese users; therefore, the descriptions were originally written in Japanese. Top and middle panels had same components; these panels were for two independent channels (the top was for the left channel, and the middle was for the right channel in stereo configuration)

2.2.2 Verification of the Algorithms

Participants
To collect data for validating our algorithm, we recruited 12 study participants, all of whom were Japanese Self-Defense Force personnel deployed on disaster relief missions following the January 12, 2010, earthquake in Haiti. All participants were native Japanese-speaking males from 30 to 59 years. The participants provided verbal consent for their voice recordings.

Participants were divided into two groups. One group consisted of participants who had been in Haiti for a long time (more than 3 months) (Group L), and the other group consisted of participants who had been in Haiti for a short time (approximately 1 week) (Group S). The participants' voice was recorded during the time that Group S participants were in Haiti. Participants in Group L had been in Haiti for at least 1 month before recording. Audio recordings were made in July and December 2010. On each recording occasion, three Group L participants and three Group S participants participated; no participants participated in both July and December.

Voice Recordings
The voices of the participants were recorded using a voice recorder ICR PS502RM (Sanyo Electric, Osaka, Japan). The recording format was a linear PCM with a sampling frequency of 44.1 kHz and a 16-bit quantization bit rate. The voice recorder was set to a low recording level and "Zoom" directivity, and all other settings (automatic volume control, peak limiter, voice-activated system, and silence segmentation) were set off to avoid processing the recorded voice by a voice recorder as much as possible.

Audio recordings were made while the study participants read a set of sentences (except one in which the participant's response depended on how they felt). Recordings were made on 6 consecutive days, twice a day, once in the morning and once in the evening. A list of sentences read by the participants is shown in Table 2.1.

Participants were instructed to hold the voice recorder at a distance of approximately 15 cm from their mouths, with the microphone facing the direction of their mouths, to perform the recording operation.

Voice Emotion Analysis
The audio recordings were analyzed after all participants returned to Japan. The audio data were transferred as electronic files from the voice recorders to a computer using ST software. After reviewing the audio files, it was determined that the audio recordings from two participants in Group L and one participant in Group S were not suitable for analysis because the volume levels were too loud and the audio waveforms were clipped beyond the maximum volume that the voice recorder could record. Therefore, the audio recordings from these participants were excluded from the analysis.

Analysis
For this study, one session was defined as a series of utterances in which all prespecified reading sentences were read. The series of utterances in a session were

Table 2.1 Manuscript of phrases read by participants

No.	Phrase	Translation
1	I-ro-ha-ni-ho-he-to	(No means like "a-b-c")
2	I-ro-ha-ni-ho-he-to	(No means like "a-b-c," repeat)
3	Watashi ha jieikan de, nihon kara kiteimasu	I belong to the Self-Defense Force and come from Japan
4	Tsukarete guttari shiteimasu	I am tired and am dead tired
5	Totemo genki desu	I am very cheerful
6	Kinou ha yoku nemuremashita	I was able to sleep well yesterday
7	Syokuyoku ga arimasu	I have an appetite
8	Okorippoi desu	I am irritable
9	Huan de ippaidesu	I am in great anxiety
10	Kokoro odayaka desu	My heart is calm
11	Kyono kibun wo iro de arawasuto {color} desu	I am {color} when I express today's feeling with a color

All phrases were in Japanese, and all participants were native Japanese speakers

divided into utterance units, which were continuous speech sounds that could be uttered in a single breath. Therefore, each session contained multiple ST utterance units, and emotion analysis using ST was performed for each utterance unit. Based on the proposed algorithm, the overall low emotional state and overall high emotional state index was calculated by combining the emotions obtained from the series of utterances.

The within-session average of the VADs calculated for all utterances in the same session for each participant was defined as the VAD of the session. One-way analysis of variance (ANOVA) was used to determine whether there were differences in the distribution of the VAD indices between Groups S and L. The ANOVA was performed using Microsoft Excel 2010.

2.3 Results

Table 2.2 shows the results of one-way ANOVA comparing the VAD indicators obtained from participants in Group S (n = 5) with those obtained from participants in Group L (n = 4).

Compared to participants in Group S, participants in Group L tended to have higher VAD-L and VAD-R and lower VAD-H. However, a one-way ANOVA revealed no significant differences in these indicators between Group S and Group L. Among the three VAD indicators, VAD-R had the largest F value. In contrast, the effect sizes η^2 were 0.1477, 0.2006, and 0.3066 for VAD-L, VAD-H, and VAD-R, respectively. Figure 2.3 shows the mean and standard deviation for each group of the normalized VAD-L, VAD-H, and VAD-R.

Table 2.2 Results of one-way analysis of variance comparing VAD indices between two participant groups

	Sum of squares	Degrees of freedom	Mean square	F-ratio	Significance level	η^2
VAD-L						
Between groups	1654	1	1654	1.213	0.3071	0.1477
Within groups	9545	7	1364			
Total	11,199	8				
VAD-H						
Between groups	558.0	1	558.0	1.756	0.2267	0.2006
Within groups	2224	7	317.7			
Total	2782	8				
VAD-R						
Between groups	204.4	1	204.4	3.096	0.1219	0.3066
Within groups	462.2	7	66.03			
Total	666.6	8				

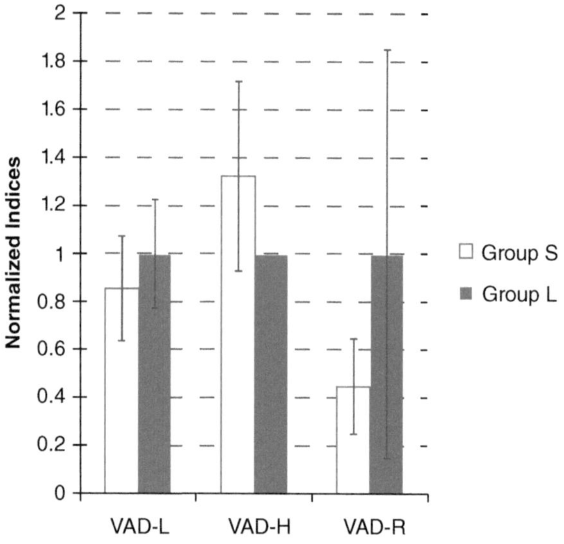

Fig 2.3 Comparison of normalized VAD indices by session between participant groups. Group S consisted of participants with a short duration of stay in the disaster area, and Group L consisted of participants with a long duration of stay in the disaster area. Indices were normalized so that the means for Group L became 1 in each index. Heights of bars show the means of the VAD indices by session for each participant group, and error bars show the standard deviations. (Modified from Mitsuyoshi et al. 2017)

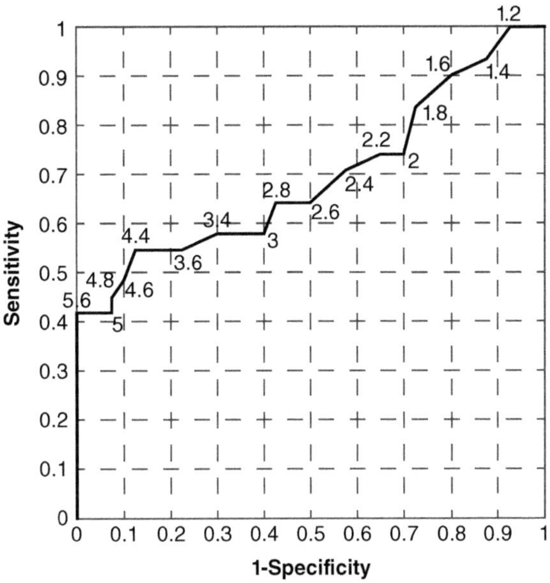

Fig 2.4 Receiver operating characteristic curve of VAD-R as a binary classifier. This curve shows performance of VAD-R index when the index is used to distinguish whether the sample is based on long-stay participants or short-stay participants. Numbers on the trace are the threshold values of VAD-R to discriminate samples from long-stay participants. (Modified from Mitsuyoshi et al. 2017)

The receiver operating characteristic (ROC) curve when the VAD-R index was used to discriminate groupings by the length of stay is shown in Fig. 2.4. The ratio of the area under the curve for this ROC curve was 0.695.

Plots of means and standard deviations obtained for each group and relative elapsed time (in half-day units) of the recording time points during the measurement period to illustrate the changes in VAD-L, VAD-H, and VAD-R over time are shown in Fig. 2.5. No significant differences were found between Groups S and L at any time point at a significance level of 0.05.

Figure 2.6 shows a comparison of the intra-individual averages of the VAD-L and VAD-H indices for each type of sentence (note that the VAD-R is calculated on a session-by-session basis, so it cannot be calculated for each sentence). The first and second sentences were averaged together because they are repetitions of the same content. No significant difference was found between groups S and L at a significance level of 0.05.

2.4 Discussion

The indices proposed in this study were designed to detect differences in affective indices between those who stayed in the disaster area for a long time (more than 3 months) (Group L) and those who stayed only for a short time (approximately 1 week) (Group S). The participants in group L tend to have higher VAD-L and lower VAD-H scores. However, the VAD indices were not significantly different between Groups L and S. In contrast, the effect size η^2 for VAD-R was 0.3066. The

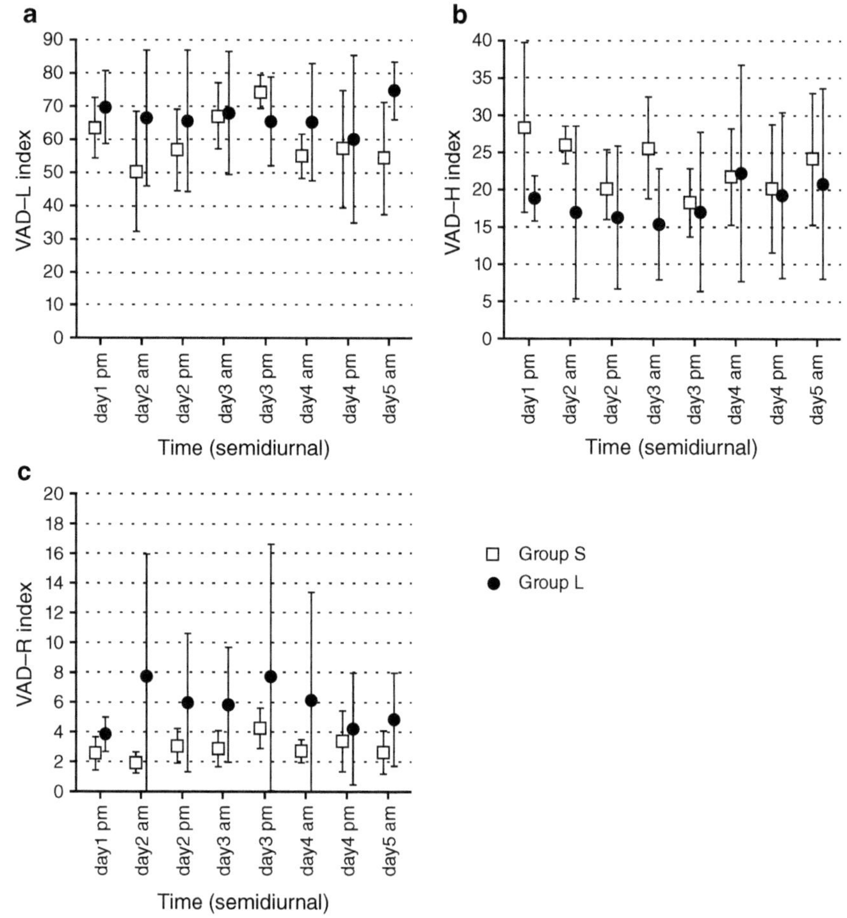

Fig. 2.5 Change in VAD indices over time. The start of the recording test was defined as the starting point of this graph (day 1). Markers show means of VAD indices by time for each participant group, and error bars show standard deviations. A, VAD-L; B, VAD-H; C, VAD-R. (Modified from Mitsuyoshi et al. 2017)

results of the analysis of emotions from the speech of these participants (Tokuno et al. 2011) indicate that there are qualitative differences in the pattern of emotional expression between long- and short-term residents; however, it is difficult to discriminate between these two groups using a single emotional index. Observing the trends in change over time, as shown in Fig. 2.5, it is clear that the change in VAD-L is a reversal of the previously reported change over time in the emotional indicators of joy and excitement (Tokuno et al. 2011). Comparing the changes over time between Groups S and L, we notice that they are switched only in the afternoon of the third day. In the sentence-by-sentence analysis, Fig. 2.6 shows that the trend of the VAD-L index is almost opposite to the trend observed for the intensity of

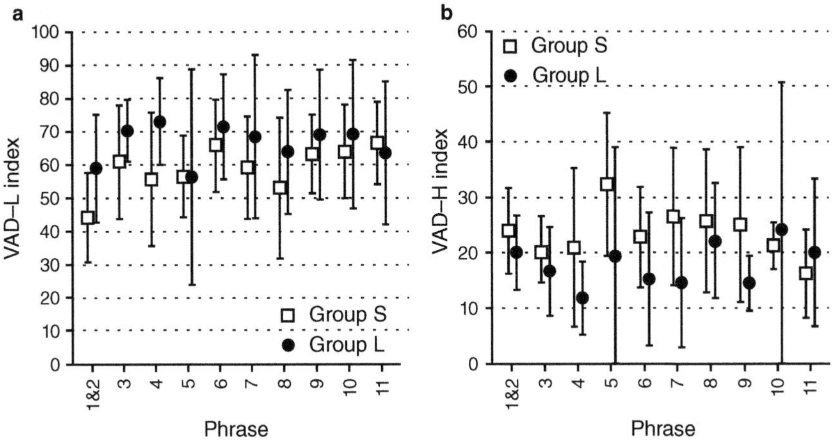

Fig. 2.6 Relationship between read phrases and VAD indices. Markers show means of VAD indices by phrase for each participant group, and error bars show standard deviations. A, VAD-L; B, VAD-H. (Modified from Mitsuyoshi et al. 2017)

excitement in particular (Tokuno et al. 2011), indicating that the intensity of the excitement index is important.

However, the ROC curve and its area under the curve indicate that applying a specific threshold to the VAD-R index is insufficient in terms of sensitivity and specificity to discriminate whether the speech data are from participants with long or short stays. In contrast, all sessions with a VAD-R greater than 5.6 are attributed to Group L participants, indicating that specificity is sufficient in areas where the VAD-R index is large.

Deployment in a disaster area is a source of stress for participating personnel, and longer stays are likely to place greater stress on participants. In contrast, long-term residents may adapt to the environment, whereas short-term residents may suffer from the stress of sudden environmental changes. The VAD indices obtained in this study suggest that the effect of the accumulated stress is more dominant. However, further research, including pre- and post-deployment measurements, is needed to assess changes over time, such as the short- and long-term effects. In addition, comparisons with those who were not deployed would provide a clearer picture of the effects of deployment.

Furthermore, as there are large individual differences in the ability to cope with stress and the actual environment experienced by dispatched personnel may not be uniform, it may not be effective to divide individuals into groups according to threshold values. In addition, it was not possible to recruit female participants in this study, and all study participants were men. Verification of whether there were differences by gender and examination of the possibility of stress assessment from the voices of female participants are considered future issues.

Because the participants in this study were sent overseas to assist with earthquake relief efforts, it was not possible to hypothesize the psychological state of the participants using biomarkers or questionnaires other than voice. Therefore, the only information that can be compared with the voice is the length of the dispatch period. The evaluation of the effectiveness of the proposed method using conventional methods remains an issue for future research.

In addition to these study items, voice of the readings of predetermined sentences were also recorded. As in the study of detecting depression from speech (Alghowinem et al. 2013), it is expected that the expression of emotion would be poorer in the reading of the written text than in spontaneous speech. Due to the difficulty of recording spontaneous utterances without a facilitator, spontaneous utterances could not be recorded in this study. Instead, the participants were able to align the content of their utterances. A comparison of speech read-out-loud and spontaneous utterances is a subject for future work.

As this was a pilot study, the number of participants was small. Further validation using data collected from a larger number of participants is required.

2.5 Conclusion

In this study, we attempted to analyze the degree of stress that a person is under based on the overall emotional state of the person who uttered the voice by applying an emotion analysis technique using voice.

By comparing data from all sessions among groups of participants who stayed for different lengths of time in a high-stress environment, we found that VAD-L, VAD-H, and VAD-R, which are indicators of the overall emotional state calculated by the algorithm proposed in this study, showed no significant differences between groups, with effect sizes η^2 of 0.1477–0.3066.

Although it was considered that the length of stay in the affected area could cause differences in VAD values due to possible effects on mental status, no psychiatrist interview or assessment of participants' mental status using existing gold standards, such as the General Health Questionnaire (Goldberg 1978), was conducted. It is expected that by examining the relationship between the VAD index proposed in this study and existing established mental health assessment methods, the usefulness of voice-based mental status assessments can be more adequately assessed.

References

Alghowinem S, Goecke R, Wagner M, Epps J, Breakspear M, Parker G (2013) Detecting depression: a comparison between spontaneous and read speech. In: Proceedings of 2013 IEEE international conference on acoustics, speech and signal processing (ICASSP 2013), Vancouver, 26–31 May 2013, pp 7547–7551

Dobashi K, Nagamine M, Shigemura J, Tsunoda T, Shimizu K, Yoshino A, Nomura S (2014) Psychological effects of disaster relief activities on Japan ground self-defense force personnel following the 2011 great east Japan earthquake. Psychiatry 77:190–198

Elfenbein HA, Ambady N (2002) On the universality and cultural specificity of emotion recognition: a meta-analysis. Psychol Bull 128:203–235

Fullerton CS, Ursano RJ, Wang L (2004) Acute stress disorder, posttraumatic stress disorder, and depression in disaster or rescue workers. Am J Psychiatry 161:1370–1376

Gao H, Yüce A, Thiran JP (2014) Detecting emotional stress from facial expressions for driving safety. In: Proceedings of 2014 IEEE international conference on image processing (ICIP 2014), Paris, 27–30 October 2014, pp 5961–5965

Goldberg DP (1978) Manual of the general health questionnaire. NFER, Windsor

Lazarus RS (1993) From psychological stress to the emotions: a history of changing outlooks. Annu Rev Psychol 44:1–21

Mitsuyoshi S (2008) Emotion recognizing method, sensibility creating method, device, and software. U.S. Patent 7 340 393

Mitsuyoshi S, Ren F, Tanaka Y, Kuroiwa S (2006) Non-verbal voice emotion analysis system. Int J Innov Comput 2:819–830

Mitsuyoshi S, Tanaka Y, Shibasaki K, Kato M, Minami T, Murata T (2007) Emotion voice analysis system connected to the human brain. In: Proceedings of international conference on natural language processing and knowledge engineering (NLP-KE), Beijing, 30 August–1 September 2007, pp 476–484

Mitsuyoshi S, Nakamura M, Omiya Y, Shinohara S, Hagiwara N, Tokuno S (2017) Mental status assessment of disaster relief personnel by vocal affect display based on voice emotion recognition. Disaster Military Med 3(1):4

Perrin MA, Di Grande L, Wheeler K, Thorpe L, Farfel M, Brackbill R (2007) Differences in PTSD prevalence and associated risk factors among World Trade Center disaster rescue and recovery workers. Am J Psychiatry 164:1385–1394

Phillips ML, Young AW, Scott SK, Calder AJ, Andrew C, Giampietro V, Williams SCR, Bullmore ET, Brammer M, Gray JA (1998) Neural responses to facial and vocal expressions of fear and disgust. Proc R Soc Lond 265:1809–1817

Raphael B, Singh B, Bradbury L, Lambert F (1984) Who helps the helpers? The effects of a disaster on the rescue workers. OMEGA—J Death Dying 14:9–20

Tian Y, Kanade T, Cohn JF (2011) Facial expression recognition. In: Li SZ, Jain A (eds) Handbook of face recognition. Springer, London, pp 487–519

Tokuno S, Tsumatori G, Shono S, Takei E, Yamamoto T, Suzuki G, Mitsuyoshi S, Shimura M (2011) Usage of emotion recognition in military health care. In: Proceedings of defense science research conference and expo, Singapore, 3–5 October 2011, pp 1–5

Chapter 3
Stress and Depressive Symptoms: Development of Mind Monitoring System (MIMOSYS)

Shuji Shinohara

3.1 Introduction

Mood disorders are a major problem in several developed countries (World Health Organization 2004), and the economic losses due to treatment costs and their impact on work are enormous (Kessler et al. 2006). Therefore, a simple method for assessing depression and stress levels is desirable. Screening methods for patients with major depressive disorder include self-administered psychological tests such as the General Health Questionnaire (GHQ) (Goldberg and Blackwell 1970; Goldberg 1978) and Beck Depression Inventory (BDI) (Beck 1961; Beck et al. 1961).

Stress checking methods using salivary (Takai et al. 2004) and blood biomarkers have been proposed (Suzuki et al. 2014). Although self-administered psychological tests are useful for early detection and diagnosis, they are limited by reporting bias, in which subjects selectively or unconsciously overestimate or underestimate certain information (Porta 2014). Stress check methods that use biomarkers in saliva or blood, while being capable of objective assessment, are limited by test costs and a burden on the subject during specimen collection, that is, low convenience.

However, with the widespread use of smartphones in recent years, pathological analysis using voice data has become popular (Arora et al. 2015; Rachuri et al. 2010; Lu et al. 2012). Speech analysis using smartphones is not only noninvasive but can also be performed easily and remotely, because it does not require dedicated equipment. The voices of depressed patients are dull, monotonous, and lifeless (Sobin and Sackeim 1997), and listeners are said to be able to perceive the illness from the patient's prosody (Darby & Hollien 1977; Yang et al. 2013). Therefore, research has been conducted on the relationship between mood disorders and speech

S. Shinohara (✉)
Division of Information Systems and Design, School of Science and Engineering, Tokyo Denki University, Hiki-gun, Saitama, Japan
e-mail: s.shinohara@mail.dendai.ac.jp

S. Tokuno, H. Nakamura (eds.), *Voice Biomarkers*,
https://doi.org/10.1007/978-981-96-3109-4_3

(Cannizzaro et al. 2004; Moore et al. 2003; Mundt et al. 2007; Vicsi et al. 2012; Taguchi et al. 2018; Wang et al. 2019).

Apart from speech pathology analysis, research on speech-based emotion recognition (Mitsuyoshi et al. 2006, 2007; Mitsuyoshi 2008) and the measurement of emotional arousal (Bone et al. 2014; Schmidt et al. 2016) have also been conducted extensively. For example, the relationship between emotional arousal and voice intensity or pitch has been reported.

Stress is known to affect emotions (Lazarus 1993). Additionally, in the fifth edition of the Diagnostic and Statistical Manual of Mental Disorders, a major depressive episode is characterized by loss of interest, happiness, sadness, and emptiness. The persistence of a depressive state accompanied by loss of interest, happiness, sadness, and emptiness is also presented (American Psychiatric Association 2013). If the process leading to depressive symptoms involves a decrease in emotions, such as joy, and an increase in emotions, such as sadness, it may be possible to detect the progression of depressive symptoms via emotion measurement. From this perspective, we focused on the relationship between mood disorders and emotions and developed a mind monitoring system (MIMOSYS), which measures the degree of mood disorders using the emotional components of speech (Shinohara et al. 2017, 2021; Higuchi et al. 2020).

3.2 Speech Emotion Recognition System

To extract emotions from speech, the speech emotion recognition software, ST Ver. 3.0 (AGI Inc., Tokyo, Japan) was used. The categories of emotion elements detected by the ST software are "anger," "joy," "sadness," "calm," and "excitement." In the ST, the strength of each emotion is expressed as an integer value ranging from "0" to "10," where "0" means that the input speech does not contain the emotion at all and 10 means that the input speech contains the emotion strongly.

The unit of speech emotion analysis by the ST software is the "utterance." This is a part of continuous speech separated by a breath. When the state of speech changes from silent to utterance, it is inferred that the speech is initiated. When the speech state continues for a certain period of time and changes to silence, it is inferred that the speech has ended. The state of silence or speech is determined from the volume, using a threshold value. The ST software uses more than 200 acoustic parameters, including the fundamental frequency, its temporal variation, and the sharpness of the rise and fall of the sound pressure, to determine the emotional category. To create the judgement algorithm, speech data from approximately 2800 people were collected, and only speech utterances for which the emotional category evaluation by others and the person in question matched were used as the training data.

3.3 Two Measures of the Extent of Mood Disorders from Emotions: Vitality and Mental Activity

We introduced two measures into MIMOSYS to describe the extent of mood disorders, vitality and mental activity; the main difference between vitality and mental activity was the duration of the measurement. Vitality is calculated from the emotional component of speech (calmness, anger, joy, sadness, excitement) over a short period, such as a single telephone conversation or hospital visit.

Conversely, mental activity is calculated from vitality data accumulated over a period of time; vitality changes occur according to the situation during measurement in the same way that blood pressure changes after exercise and at rest. In the same way that long-term monitoring provides an accurate picture of hypertension, MIMOSYS aims to provide a more accurate picture of mood disorders by introducing mental activity.

3.4 Collection of Voice Data

We used speech data from healthy subjects and outpatients attending hospitals with major depression to develop an algorithm to calculate vitality and mental activity based on emotions. The audio of the healthy subjects was acquired between February and mid-May 2015. During the acquisition period, the participants did not visit medical facilities for mood-related illnesses and worked normally. Audio acquisition was conducted every few days, with 14 standardized phrases read twice each time. Voice recordings were performed in a quiet environment with minimal background noise.

The patient was acquired between August 2013 and October 2014. The patients' audio recordings were conversations with the doctor during consultation. Overlaps in speech by the doctor and background noise were manually removed.

Table 3.1 lists the participant information by group. It should be noted that the number of data is higher than the number of participants because data were collected multiple times on different days from the same participants. The mean number of data collected per healthy participant ± standard deviation (SD) was 24.4 ± 33.3 for men and 6.3 ± 6.1 for women. For depressed patients, this was

Table 3.1 Participant information for voice collection experiments (for algorithm creation)

Group	Sex	Number of participants			Mean age	Number of data		
Healthy	Male	9	13	22	42.9 ± 5.6	220	245	303
	Female	4			33.3 ± 15.4	25		
Patient	Male	4	9		54.0 ± 12.0	24	58	
	Female	5			49.4 ± 15.4	34		

6.0 ± 2.9 for men and 6.8 ± 3.2 for women. Based on these collected data, an algorithm was developed to calculate vitality and mental activity.

Regarding the abovementioned acquired speech, the speech of a healthy person is a recording of regular phrase speech. Conversely, the voice of the patient is a recording of a conversation with a doctor, that is, free speech, and the form of speech differs between a healthy person and the patient. The recording locations were different. Therefore, to unify the speech form and recording environment, data for the algorithm validation were collected at a university hospital.

The speech recordings of canned phrases were collected from outpatients with major depression between December 2015 and June 2016. The 17 standardized Japanese phrases used for the recordings are listed in Table 3.2. During voice collection, specialists assessed the patients' depression severity using the Hamilton Depression Rating Scale (HAM-D) (Hamilton 1967), which is a rating of the characteristic items of depression symptoms by doctors and other specialists and can objectively quantify an individual's depressive state.

For the voices of healthy subjects, voice recordings were made in mid-December 2016 in the same consultation room as the patient, reading the same standardized phrases as the patient. However, the HAM-D has not been used to assess the severity of depression in healthy subjects.

Table 3.3 presents information on the participants in the voice collection experiment for algorithm validation. The number of healthy participants and their voice

Table 3.2 Seventeen canned phrases for recording

No.	Phrase in Japanese	Purpose (meaning)
1	I-ro-ha-ni-ho-he-to	Nonemotional (no meaning, like "a-b-c")
2	Honjitsu ha seiten nari	Nonemotional (It is fine today)
3	Tsurezurenaru mama ni	Nonemotional (Having nothing to do)
4	Wagahai ha neko dearu	Nonemotional (I am a cat)
5	Mukashi aru tokoro ni	Nonemotional (Once upon a time, there lived)
6	a-i-u-e-o	Check pronunciation of vowel sounds (no meaning like "a-b-c")
7	Ga-gi-gu-ge-go	Check sonant pronunciation (no meaning, like "a-b-c")
8	Ra-ri-ru-re-ro	Check liquid sound pronunciation (no meaning, like "a-b-c")
9	Pa-pi-pu-pe-po	Check p-sound pronunciation (no meaning, like "a-b-c")
10	Omoeba tooku he kita monda	Nonemotional (While thinking, I have come far)
11	Garapagosu shotou	Check pronunciation (Galápagos Islands)
12	Tsukarete guttari shiteimasu.	Emotional (I am tired/dead tired)
13	Totemo genki desu	Emotional (I am very cheerful)
14	Kinou ha yoku nemuremashita	Emotional (I was able to sleep well yesterday)
15	Shokuyoku ga arimasu	Emotional (I have an appetite)
16	Okorippoi desu	Emotional (I am irritable)
17	Kokoroga odayaka desu	Emotional (My heart is calm)

Table 3.3 Participant information for voice collection experiments (for algorithm validation)

Group	Sex	Number of participants			Mean age	Number of data		
Healthy	Male	10	14	44	42.7 ± 6.0	10	14	60
	Female	4			35.0 ± 14.4	4		
Patient	Male	19	30		43.7 ± 11.0	34	46	
	Female	11			53.9 ± 8.2	12		

data for validation is the same as that of the healthy participants for validation because voice data were collected only once per person. For the patients, some participants had more than one data collection: seven participants had two data collections, three had three data collections, and one had four data collections. From the remaining 19 participants, data were acquired only once. The recording format of the abovementioned audio was linear PCM, with a sampling frequency of 11025 Hz and a quantization bit rate of 16 bits.

3.5 Algorithm for Calculating Vitality and Mental Activity

3.5.1 Vitality Calculation Algorithm

To calculate vitality from the emotional component, we introduced two new indicators: vivacity and relaxation. To define these indicators, we used four of the five indicators output by the ST: calm, joy, sadness, and excitement.

In the fifth edition of the Diagnostic and Statistical Manual of Mental Disorders, the characteristics of a major depressive episode include loss of interest and happiness and a persistent state of depression with sadness and emptiness (American Psychiatric Association 2013). Conversely, if the joyful component is greater than sadness in the emotion, it is considered a good mood state. In this context, the vivacity of an utterance is defined as follows:

$$\text{vivacity} = \frac{\text{joy}}{\text{joy} + \text{sorrow}} \tag{3.1}$$

where joy and sorrow represent the strengths of the joy and sorrow components detected in the utterance using ST, respectively. Because the denominator of Eq. (3.1) is the sum of the strengths of joy and sorrow and the numerator is the strength of joy, the greater the strength of joy relative to the strength of sorrow, the greater the vivacity value.

Stress and tension are major factors in mood disorders. Conversely, a relaxed state is considered a good mental state. From this perspective, the degree of relaxation derived from the emotional component of an utterance is defined as

$$\text{relaxation} = \frac{\text{calm}}{\text{calm} + \text{excitement}} \tag{3.2}$$

Here, calm and excitement represent the strength of the calm and excitement components detected from the utterance using the ST, respectively. In other words, the level of relaxation increases as the calm component of emotion increases and the excitement component decreases.

In ST, the recorded speech was first divided into utterances, and the strength of each emotion for each utterance was expressed as an integer value between 0 and 10. Therefore, the vivacity and relaxation degrees are real numbers in the range of 0.0–1.0. The vivacity and relaxation defined above are calculated for each utterance. Furthermore, the average of the vivacity and relaxation of all utterances in the acquired speech was defined as the vivacity and relaxation of the entire acquired speech, respectively.

Vitality was calculated as the weighted average of vivacity and relaxation. Figure 3.1 shows a scatter diagram of the vivacity and relaxation calculated from the data for algorithm creation. Based on the straight lines in the diagram, the vitality of each acquired voice was defined as follows:

$$\text{vitality} = 0.60 \times \text{vivacity} + 0.40 \times \text{relaxation} \tag{3.3}$$

3.5.2 *Mental Activity Calculation Algorithm*

Vitality was calculated from audio recordings obtained over a short period of time, such as a single examination or consultation. Therefore, depending on the mood of the experimental participant during measurement, vitality may be low, even in healthy people, or conversely high in patients. To compensate for this weakness, the mental activity was calculated from long-term trends in vitality.

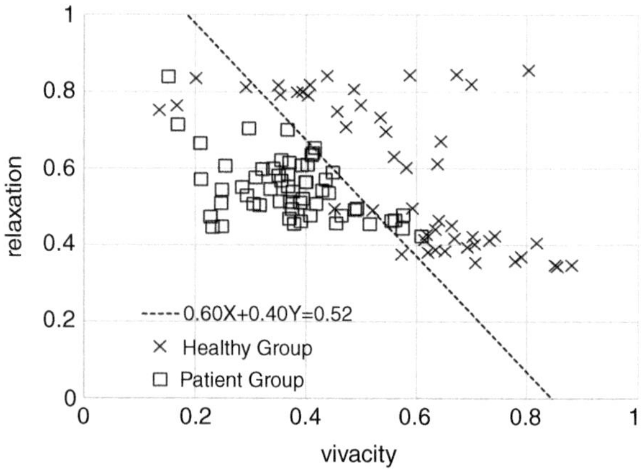

Fig. 3.1 Scatterplot of the degree of vivacity and relaxation. Data are plotted per recorded voice data. There are 50 data for the 13 healthy subjects group and 58 data for the 9 patient groups. The straight line illustrated (0.60X + 0.40Y = 0.52) separates the healthy and patient groups. (Modified from Shinohara et al. 2021)

In the fifth edition of the Diagnostic and Statistical Manual of Mental Disorders published by the American Psychiatric Association, depression is defined as a condition that includes two symptoms, namely, a "depressed mood" and "markedly diminished interest and pleasure," and three or more of seven symptoms, including "insomnia or excessive sleep" and "repetitive thoughts about death," lasting more than 2 weeks.

In other words, depression is defined as a state of feeling depressed or blocked up, feeling sad, or not being happy about a happy event for 2 or more weeks. Therefore, the period for calculating mental activity was set to 2 weeks.

Specifically, the average value ($\overline{Vitality}$) of the 2 weeks of accumulated vitality for each individual was calculated to represent a 2-week trend in vitality. Furthermore, it was decided to judge mental activity as low if vitality fluctuated slightly and stagnated at a low value. To realize this, the standard deviation of vitality (vitality SD) was introduced as an indicator of the extent to which the vitality of each utterance in the recorded speech fluctuated. The mean value ($\overline{Vitality\mathrm{SD}}$) of the accumulated vitality, SD, for each individual was then calculated.

Figure 3.2 shows a scatterplot of the mean vitality and mean vitality standard deviation for each participant, calculated from the data for algorithm creation. In the figure, 1 point is plotted for each subject, and the number of data points is 22 in total, for the 13 healthy subjects group and 9 patients group. The figure is accompanied by a straight line (0.75X + 0.25Y = 0.426) separating the healthy and patient groups. Based on this straight line, mental activity was defined as follows: using the mean value of vitality and the mean value of the standard deviation of vitality.

$$\mathrm{mental\_activity} = 0.75 \times \overline{\mathrm{vitality}} + 0.25 \times \overline{\mathrm{vitalitySD}} \tag{3.4}$$

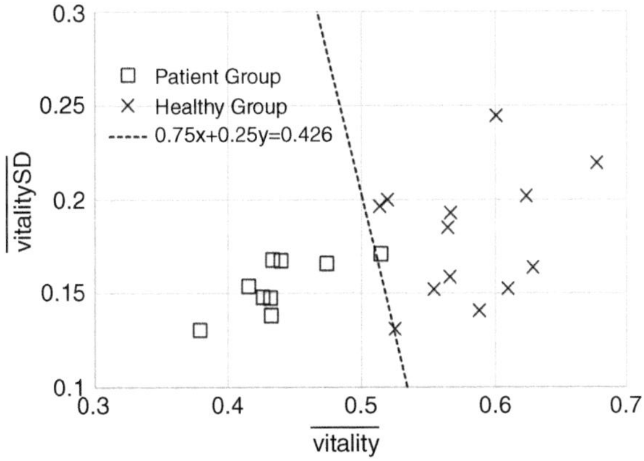

Fig. 3.2 Scatterplot of the vitality mean and vitality standard deviation mean for each participant ($N = 22$). (Modified from Shinohara et al. 2021)

3.6 Evaluation

3.6.1 Evaluation Method

The data for the algorithm validation presented in Table 3.3 were used as assessment data, following the definition of Zimmerman et al. (2013). The data of the patient group were divided into two groups based on the HAM-D score: no depression (≤7) and depression (≥8). The vitality of these two groups and that of the healthy groups were compared.

The accuracy of the vitality classification was assessed by the *P*-value from the Tukey–Kramer test, as well as by the AUC, sensitivity, and specificity. Additionally, the power of the test and effect size using Cohen's d were calculated. For all analyses, the significance level was set at $P < 0.05$.

The following analyses were performed using the statistical software R (version 3.6.1; 2019-07-05) (The Comprehensive R Archive Network 2020), unless otherwise specified.

The R packages of epi version 2.41 for AUC calculation, multcomp version 1.4.16 for the Tukey–Kramer test, effsize version 0.8.1 for Cohen's d calculation, and pwr version 1.3.0 for sample size estimation were used. The operating system was Windows 10.

3.6.2 HAM-D Score

The mean HAM-D scores of the two groups of patients are listed in Table 3.4. The number of participants in each group was 11 men and 8 women in the no depression group and 8 men and 3 women in the depression group. The number of participants in each group was as follows: no depression group, 15 males and 9 females; depression group, 19 males and 3 females.

Table 3.4 Average value of Hamilton Rating Scale for Depression (HAM-D) score for each group

Group	Sex	Number of data		Mean HAM-D score ± SD	
No depression (HAM-D ≤ 7)	Male	15	24	3.6 ± 2.4	3.1 ± 2.3
	Female	9		2.3 ± 2.1	
Depression (HAM-D ≥ 8)	Male	19	22	17.2 ± 7.4	16.1 ± 7.4
	Female	3		9.7 ± 2.9	

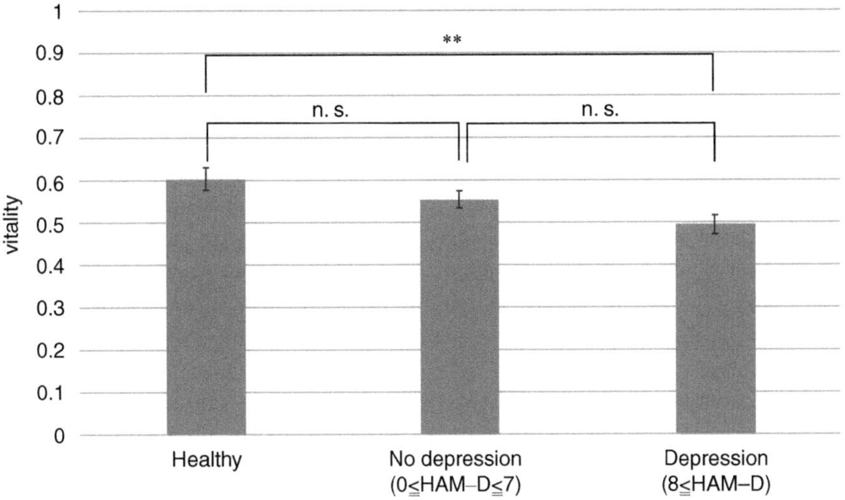

Fig. 3.3 Comparison of vitality for each group. Error bars represent standard error. ** ($p < 0.01$), *n.s.* not significant. *HAM-D* Hamilton Rating Scale for Depression. (Modified from Shinohara et al. 2021)

3.6.3 *Vitality Performance*

The vitality performance was evaluated using the data for the algorithm validation presented in Table 3.3. First, a significant negative correlation was found between the HAM-D score and vitality for the 46 data points from the patient group ($r = -0.33$, $n = 46$, $p < 0.05$).

Figure 3.3 then shows a comparison of the vitality scores of the healthy, no depression, and depressed groups. The mean vitality for each group was 0.60 ± 0.027 ($n = 14$), 0.55 ± 0.020 ($n = 24$), and 0.49 ± 0.022 ($n = 22$), respectively. The Tukey–Kramer test showed a significant difference between the healthy and depressed groups ($p = 0.0085$). The effect size for vitality between the healthy and depressed patients was 1.03. When this value was used as the effect size and the significance level was set at 0.05, the power of the test was 0.84. This value is greater than 0.8, indicating that the power of the test is large.

However, when the number of data points for the depression group was 22, with a power of 0.8, significance level of 0.05, and effect size of 1.03, the required sample size for the healthy group was 12.13. In this study, the number of data points for the healthy group was 14, which is slightly higher. The AUC of the ROC curve, sensitivity, and specificity was used to assess the discriminative performance of vitality. For the discrimination performance of the healthy and depressed groups, the AUC was 0.76, whereas the sensitivity and specificity were 0.93 and 0.55, respectively.

3.7 Discussion and Conclusions

We developed MIMOSYS to measure the degree of mood disorders using the emotional component of speech. We proposed two indicators of the degree of mood disorder: vitality, based on short-term speech data, and mental activity, calculated from long-term speech data. A significant negative correlation was observed between the vitality and HAM-D scores. As shown in Fig. 3.3, vitality can be used to discriminate speech data from healthy and depressed patients with a high accuracy. However, no significant differences were observed between the no depression group, which had few depressive symptoms, even among depressed outpatients and the healthy group. This suggests the possibility of measuring the treatment effects using vitality.

If the correlation between the HAM-D score and vitality can be further improved, it could be used in the future to assist doctors in diagnosis. If MIMOSYS can be implemented on smartphones, vitality and mental activity can be monitored daily, which could be used to encourage people to go to hospitals before depression or in the early stages of depression. This could lead to a reduction in economic losses from treatment costs and disruptions to work. It was not possible to evaluate mental activity performance because it was not possible to continuously obtain a large amount of data from each subject. The evaluation of mental activity is presented in Chaps. 4 and 5.

References

American Psychiatric Association (2013) Diagnostic and statistical manual of mental disorders, 5th edn. Arlington, American Psychiatric Association. https://doi.org/10.1176/appi.books.9780890425596

Arora S, Venkataraman V, Zhan A, Donohue S, Biglan KM, Dorsey ER, Little MA (2015) Detecting and monitoring the symptoms of Parkinson's disease using smartphones: a pilot study. Parkinsonism Relat Disord 21(6):650–653. https://doi.org/10.1016/j.parkreldis.2015.02.026

Beck AT (1961) A systematic investigation of depression. Compr Psychiatry 2(3):163–170. https://doi.org/10.1016/S0010-440X(61)80020-5

Beck AT, Ward CH, Mendelson M, Mock J, Erbaugh J (1961) An inventory for measuring depression. Arch Gen Psychiatry 4(6):561–571. https://doi.org/10.1001/archpsyc.1961.01710120031004

Bone D, Lee CC, Narayanan S (2014) Robust unsupervised arousal rating: a rule-based framework with knowledge-inspired vocal features. IEEE Trans Affect Comput 5:201–213. https://doi.org/10.1109/TAFFC.2014.2326393

Cannizzaro M, Harel B, Reilly N, Chappell P, Snyder PJ (2004) Voice acoustical measurement of the severity of major depression. Brain Cogn 56(1):30–35. https://doi.org/10.1016/j.bandc.2004.05.003

Darby JK, Hollien H (1977) Vocal and speech patterns of depressive patients. Folia Phoniatr Logop 29:279–291

Goldberg D (1978) Manual of the general health questionnaire. Windsor, NFER Nelson

Goldberg DP, Blackwell B (1970) Psychiatric illness in general practice: a detailed study using a new method of case identification. Br Med J 2(5707):439–443. https://doi.org/10.1136/bmj.2.5707.439

Hamilton MA (1967) Development of a rating scale for primary depressive illness. Br J Soc Clin Psychol 6(4):278–296. https://doi.org/10.1111/j.2044-8260.1967.tb00530.x
Higuchi M, Nakamura M, Shinohara S, Omiya Y, Takano T, Mitsuyoshi S, Tokuno S (2020) Effectiveness of a voice-based mental health evaluation system for mobile devices: prospective study. JMIR Formative Res 4(7):e16455. https://doi.org/10.2196/16455
Kessler RC, Akiskal HS, Ames M, Birnbaum H, Greenberg P, Hirschfeld RMA, Jin R, Merikangas KR, Simon GE, Wang PS (2006) Prevalence and effects of mood disorders on work performance in a nationally representative sample of U.S. workers. Am J Psychiatry 163(9):1561–1568. https://doi.org/10.1176/ajp.2006.163.9.1561
Lazarus RS (1993) From psychological stress to the emotions: a history of changing outlooks. Annu Rev Psychol 44(1):1–22. https://doi.org/10.1146/annurev.ps.44.020193.000245
Lu H, Frauendorfer D, Rabbi M, Mast MS, Chittaranjan GT, Campbell AT, Gatica-Perez D, Choudhury T (2012) Stresssense: detecting stress in unconstrained acoustic environments using smartphones. In: Proceedings of the 2012 ACM conference on ubiquitous computing, September 5. ACM, pp 351–360. https://doi.org/10.1145/2370216.2370270
Mitsuyoshi S (2008) Inventor; Advanced Generation Interface Inc, assignee. Emotion recognizing method, sensibility creating method, device, and software. United States patent US 7, 340, 393
Mitsuyoshi S, Ren F, Tanaka Y, Kuroiwa S (2006) Non-verbal voice emotion analysis system. Int J ICIC 2(4):819–830
Mitsuyoshi S, Shibasaki K, Tanaka Y, Kato M, Murata T, Minami T, Yagura H, Ren F (2007) Emotion voice analysis system connected to the human brain. In: 2007 international conference on natural language processing and knowledge engineering, Beijing, China, 2007 IEEE, pp 476–484. https://doi.org/10.1109/NLPKE.2007.4368074
Moore E, Clements M, Peifer J, Weisser L (2003) Analysis of prosodic variation in speech for clinical depression. In: Proceedings of the 25th annual international conference of the IEEE engineering in medicine and biology society, Cancun, Mexico 2003 September 17. IEEE IEEE Cat. No. 03CH37439, vol 3, pp 2925–2928. https://doi.org/10.1109/IEMBS.2003.1280531
Mundt JC, Snyder PJ, Cannizzaro MS, Chappie K, Geralts DS (2007) Voice acoustic measures of depression severity and treatment response collected via interactive voice response (IVR) technology. J Neurolinguistics 20(1):50–64. https://doi.org/10.1016/j.jneuroling.2006.04.001
Porta MA (2014) Dictionary of epidemiology, 6th edn. Oxford University Press, New York
Rachuri KK, Musolesi M, Mascolo C, Rentfrow PJ, Longworth C, Aucinas A (2010) EmotionSense: a mobile phones based adaptive platform for experimental social psychology research. In: Proceedings of the 12th ACM international conference on Ubiquitous computing, September 26. ACM, pp 281–290. https://doi.org/10.1145/1864349.1864393
Schmidt J, Janse E, Scharenborg O (2016) Perception of emotion in conversational speech by younger and older listeners. Front Psychol 7:781. https://doi.org/10.3389/fpsyg.2016.00781
Shinohara S, Omiya Y, Hagiwara N, Nakamura M, Higuchi M, Kirita T, Takano T, Mitsuyoshi S, Tokuno S (2017) Case studies of utilization of the mind monitoring system (MIMOSYS) using voice and its future prospects. ESMS J 7(1):7–12
Shinohara S, Nakamura M, Omiya Y, Higuchi M, Hagiwara N, Mitsuyoshi S, Toda H, Saito T, Tanichi M, Yoshino A, Tokuno S (2021) Depressive mood assessment method based on emotion level derived from voice: comparison of voice features of individuals with major depressive disorders and healthy controls. Int J Environ Res Public Health 18(10):5435. https://doi.org/10.3390/ijerph18105435
Sobin C, Sackeim HA (1997) Psychomotor symptoms of depression. Am J Psychiatry 154:4–17
Suzuki G, Tokuno S, Nibuya M, Ishida T, Yamamoto T, Mukai Y, Mitani K, Tsumatori G, Scott D, Shimizu K (2014) Decreased plasma brain-derived neurotrophic factor and vascular endothelial growth factor concentrations during military training. PLoS One 9(2):e89455:1–e89455:8. https://doi.org/10.1371/journal.pone.0089455
Taguchi T et al (2018) Major depressive disorder discrimination using vocal acoustic features. J Affect Disord 225:214–220. https://doi.org/10.1016/j.jad.2017.08.038
Takai N, Yamaguchi M, Aragaki T, Eto K, Uchihashi K, Nishikawa Y (2004) Effect of psychological stress on the salivary cortisol and amylase levels in healthy young adults. Arch Oral Biol 49(12):963–968. https://doi.org/10.1016/j.archoralbio.2004.06.007

The Comprehensive R Archive Network. Available online: cran.r-project.org/. Accessed 15 July 2020
Vicsi K, Sztahó D, Kiss G (2012) Examination of the sensitivity of acoustic-phonetic parameters of speech to depression. In: 2012 IEEE 3rd international conference on cognitive info communications (CogInfoCom), Kosice, Slovakia, 2012 December 2. IEEE, pp 511–515. https://doi.org/10.1109/CogInfoCom.2012.6422035
Wang J, Zhang L, Liu T, Pan W, Hu B, Zhu T (2019) Acoustic differences between healthy and depressed people: a cross-situation study. BMC Psychiatry 19(1):300
World Health Organization (2004) The global burden of disease: 2004 update. WHO Press, Geneva, pp 46–49
Yang Y, Fairbairn C, Cohn JF (2013) Detecting depression severity from vocal prosody. IEEE Trans Affect Comput 4:142–150. https://doi.org/10.1109/T-AFFC.2012.38
Zimmerman M, Martinez JH, Young D, Chelminski I, Dalrymple K (2013) Severity classification on the Hamilton depression rating scale. J Affect Disord 150(2):384–388. https://doi.org/10.1016/j.jad.2013.04.028

Chapter 4
Stress and Depressive Symptoms: Validation of MIMOSYS (Engineering)

Takeshi Takano

4.1 Introduction

The most effective use of MIMOSYS, which can estimate mental health status from voice, is its implementation as an application that can continuously record daily. The recent proliferation of smartphones has made it possible to easily perform everything, from voice acquisition to advanced signal processing, without special devices. In addition to smartphones, MIMOSYS can also be implemented in smart homes and vehicles, provided they can acquire audio and run in programmable devices.

However, the implementation of this technology in these devices may be severely affected by the characteristics of onboard microphones and background noise. For example, in applications that acquire voice over a phone, the voice is compressed to reduce the amount of data transmission, and the changes in acoustic characteristics during the conversion process raises a concern. In addition, there is concern that ambient noise will be added to the target voice in outdoor applications during the daytime. Furthermore, the application's design may limit the recording methods and may need to accommodate users who speak different languages.

We validate MIMOSYS from an engineering perspective, to verify its applications and limitations.

T. Takano (✉)
Department of Pharmacology, School of Medicine, UT Health San Antonio, San Antonio, TX, USA
e-mail: takanot@uthscsa.edu

S. Tokuno, H. Nakamura (eds.), *Voice Biomarkers*,
https://doi.org/10.1007/978-981-96-3109-4_4

4.2 Differences in Sex and Age

It is known that the properties of voice vary with sex and age, and this fact has been reported by various previous studies. Accordingly, we investigated the impact of these voice characteristics on MIMOSYS.

We collected voice and BDI scores from 36 men and 45 women aged ≥18 years and older with no pre-existing medical conditions for 2 weeks. The number of people per age category is presented in Table 4.1, and the mean values of the age, BDI, vitality, and mental activity for each sex are presented in Table 4.2. We converted these voices to vitality and mental activity using MIMOSYS and then compared the scores to BDIs.

Figure 4.1 presents the scatterplot of age and vitality, while Fig. 4.2 illustrates the scatterplot of the age of each subject and mental activity. The correlation coefficients are presented in Table 4.3.

The obtained results exhibited no difference between the indices for men and women and no correlation between age, vitality, and mental activity. These results indicate that MIMOSYS is not affected by sex or age.

4.3 Differences in Recording Methods

When deploying MIMOSYS in an application, we may be faced with the challenge of choosing which spontaneous speech or fixed-phrase speech recording method to use. This is owing to the assumption that the output will change between spontaneous speech, which is more likely to express emotions, and fixed-phrase speech, which is less likely to exhibit such behavior. In addition, it is important to consider that the timing of free speech acquisition is limited and that the recorded voice may contain sensitive information such as personal information. Therefore, to verify the differences in MIMOSYS characteristics between spontaneous and fixed-phrase speeches, we developed a smartphone application that can record both methods and

Table 4.1 Number of subjects by age group

Age group	Male	Female
18–19	2	4
20–24	1	3
25–29	6	4
30–34	6	3
35–39	4	6
40–44	3	3
45–49	7	1
50–54	4	10
55–59	2	7
60–64	1	5

Table 4.2 Age and average value of each indicator by sex

	Male (n = 36)	Female (n = 45)
Age	39.1(SD = 11.6)	43.0 (SD = 14.0)
BDI	3.2 (SE = 0.48)	3.4 (SE = 0.49)
Vitality	41.1 (SE = 1.7)	40.1 (SE = 1.2)
Mental activity	53.9 (SE = 2.1)	52.0 (SE = 1.3)

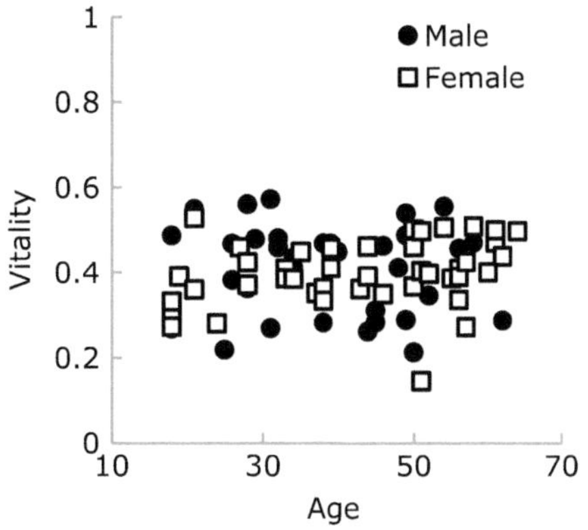

Fig. 4.1 Scatterplot of age and vitality

compared the frequency of acquiring MIMOSYS output values. This application had two approaches to acquiring voice records: automatically acquiring spontaneous speech triggered by incoming and outgoing calls and acquiring fixed-phrase speech by pressing the button on the recording screen and reading out the displayed text. The first approach is referred to as "auto-recording" and the second way as "manual recording." We installed this app on the smartphones of 47 subjects and instructed them to analyze MIMOSYS every day.

First, we surveyed to verify the method that was more likely to be used by comparing the auto-recording and manual recording usage rates. The usage rates were calculated by dividing the number of subjects recorded at least once a day by the total number of subjects. Figure 4.3 illustrates the changes in the usage rates during the experimental period. The average rates for the first and second halves of the voice collection period are presented in Table 4.4. These results can be attributed to two factors. In the first half, the advantage of manual recording was more significant than that of auto-recording because it can be used at any time. However, the usage rate decreased to less than that of the auto-recording in the second half because it requires action.

Next, we compared the difference between the MIMOSYS outputs of the auto-recording and manual recording. According to a study on emotions and vitality calculated by MIMOSYS in two approaches, it was inferred that the emotions of calm and sorrow tended to appear more strongly in manual recordings, while the emotions of anger, joy, and excitement were stronger in auto recordings (Fig. 4.4). Consequently, the distribution of the vitality of auto recordings was also higher than that of manual recordings.

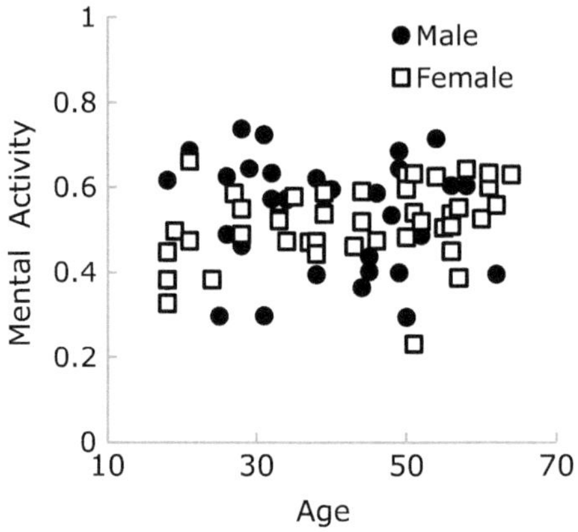

Fig. 4.2 Scatterplot of age and mental activity

Table 4.3 Correlation between age and each indicator

	Correlation coefficient
Age vs vitality	0.11
Age vs mental activity	0.13

From these results, we obtain the following three findings:

1. Auto recording is effective for continuous daily monitoring.
2. Manual recording exhibits a significant decrease in utilization over time.
3. Vitality of manual recordings is inferior to that of auto recordings.

Hence, the MIMOSYS application should be designed considering these results.

4.4 Effect of Audio Format

Recently, as semiconductors have become more powerful, various devices are being developed to collect voice data. However, the performance of these devices, their operating systems, application limitations, and communication methods do not allow for a free choice of voice formats. In addition, the primary objective of the recording function of most devices is to transmit voice information, and there is a concern that devices that adopt lossy compression methods and communications may lack the voice components necessary for MIMOSYS analysis.

By converting the collected speech into various speech formats, converting it back to the original format, and comparing the obtained results to the original sound, we investigated the impact of the speech format on the results of the MIMOSYS analysis.

The sampling rate is the most common problem encountered when analyzing MIMOSYS in applications. The sensibility technology (ST), which is the basis of

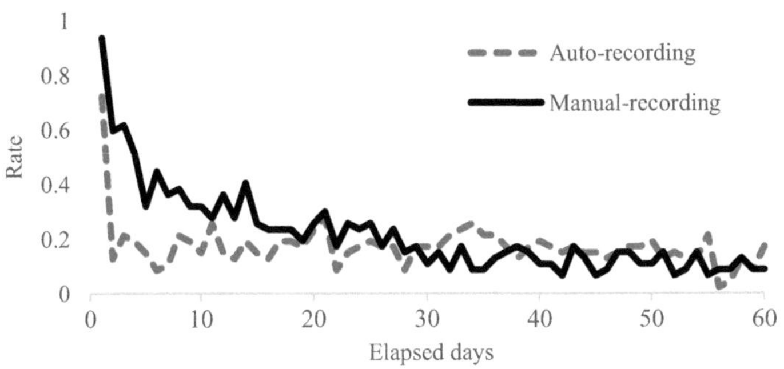

Fig. 4.3 Trends in recording rate

Table 4.4 Comparison of recording rates between first and second half

	First half	Second half	t-test
Method	Rate	Rate	(*p*-value)
Auto-recording	0.19	0.16	0.218 n. s
Manual recording	0.32	0.11	1.08E-07***
			(***$p < 0.01$)

MIMOSYS, was developed to accept a linear pulse code modulation (PCM) format with a bit depth and sampling rate of 16 bits and 11.025 kHz (1 ch), respectively. However, ST has been recently developed to input at 8 kHz. However, several recordings have been made at sampling rates of 8 kHz, 16 kHz, and 48 kHz, with 8 kHz as the axis. Among these, the 8-kHz sampling is less frequent than 11.025-kHz sampling, thereby resulting in missing information in high-frequency components and making it impossible to interpolate from the preceding and following data. To evaluate the degree of missing information at 8 kHz, we compared the results of the MIMOSYS analysis of an original 11.025 kHz sound source and that of a voice that was downsampled to 8 kHz and then upsampled to 11.025 kHz, thereby missing the high-frequency components (Hagiwara et al. 2017).

A correlation coefficient of 0.871 was deduced between the original pressure before and after resampling, thus suggesting the effectiveness of upsampling the speech resampled at 8 kHz and analyzing it via MIMOSYS.

Next, we compared the analysis results of decoded speech encoded in μ-law, A-law, G.726, and G.723.1, which were used in telephone lines, with the analysis results of the original speech (Hagiwara et al. 2017). G.711, in which μ-law and A-law are defined, is a standard for exchanging voice over ISDN; however, μ-law is primarily used in the United States and Japan, while A-law is adopted in the EU. The format employed to input MIMOSYS is linear PCM, which records values proportional to sound pressure. However, to reduce the volume of information transmitted over telephone lines, the ITU-T defines various data

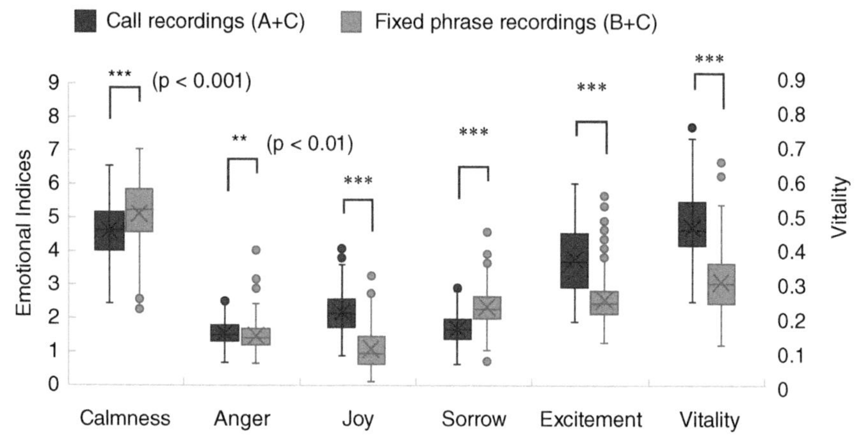

Fig. 4.4 Distribution of emotions and vitality by recording method

Table 4.5 Correlation of vitality between coding standards for voice communication and MIMOSYS standard format (Hagiwara et al. 2017)

	11.025-kHz Linear PCM	8-kHz Linear PCM
8-kHz Linear PCM	0.871	–
G.711Mu (μ-law)	0.868	0.975
G.711 (A-law)	0.865	0.974
G.726 (ADPCM)	0.865	0.969
G.723.1 (MPC-MLQ)	0.849	0.948

formats. For example, the μ-law is a format in which the sound pressure is proportional to the sound pressure. It records sound pressure in logarithmic form to achieve a large dynamic range even with a small bit depth. However, linear PCM has the disadvantage of lacking information on minute changes in the sound pressure within the recorded loud sound. Because each encoding method has its advantages and disadvantages, we evaluated their effects on the analysis results. Accordingly, correlation coefficients of 0.868, 0.865, 0.865, and 0.849 were obtained. Further analysis and comparison with the results for the 8-kHz resampled speech studied earlier yielded correlation coefficients of 0.975, 0.974, 0.969, and 0.948, respectively. Because telephone speech is transmitted after downsampling to 8 kHz, it is inevitably affected by resampling. However, the change in the MIMOSYS results was significantly more attributable to resampling than to encoding itself. Table 4.5 presents a summary of these results.

Table 4.6 Correlation of vitality between audio coding standard for music and MIMOSYS standard format

	11.025-kHz Linear PCM
AAC (MPEG-2)	0.975
MP3 (MPEG-1 layer 3)	0.961
WMA	0.965

Another study reported the results of encoding and decoding AAC, MP3, and WMA formats commonly used in music, which obtained correlation coefficients of 0.975, 0.961, and 0.965, respectively (Table 4.6).

These results demonstrate the effectiveness of MIMOSYS, even for speech sampled at 8 kHz and recorded with various encodings.

4.5 Effects of Noise Environment

When using MIMOSYS as an application, it is rare to record in an ideal quiet environment in actual usage scenarios, and the audio is recorded with noise that more or less differs from the target audio. The amount of noise in the recorded audio is indicated by the signal-to-noise ratio (SNR). An example is provided to facilitate the understanding of the SNR. The sound pressures of a normal conversation and quiet office are approximately 60 dB and 50 dB, respectively. Hence, an SNR of 10 dB represents the ratio of the noise level of a conversation in a quiet office. Consequently, speech is effortless in such an environment. However, the background noise level of −20 dB SNR is 80 dB, corresponding to a noisy environment such as a construction site. In such an environment, we would not be able to hear the voice of another person; hence, the need to shout is unavoidable.

We utilized the speech corpus CENSREC-1-C to investigate the effect of the MIMOSYS output by synthesizing eight types of noise, adjusted from −5 to 20 dB for speech: subway, babble noise, car cabin, exhibition hall, restaurant, nearby street, airport, and station (Higuchi et al. 2018).

The obtained results are presented in Fig. 4.5. From Fig. 4.5, at SNRs of 20 dB and 15 dB, the original pressure tends to decrease compared to the original sound; however, the changing trend alters significantly from SNR 10. This is because the number of utterances detected for analysis decreases as the noise level increases, and the analysis interval changed, as illustrated in Fig. 4.6. When the accuracy of the MIMOSYS speech detection in the presence of noise improves in the future, it may become possible to mitigate the effects of noise by applying appropriate filtering to speech containing noise and taking advantage of these findings.

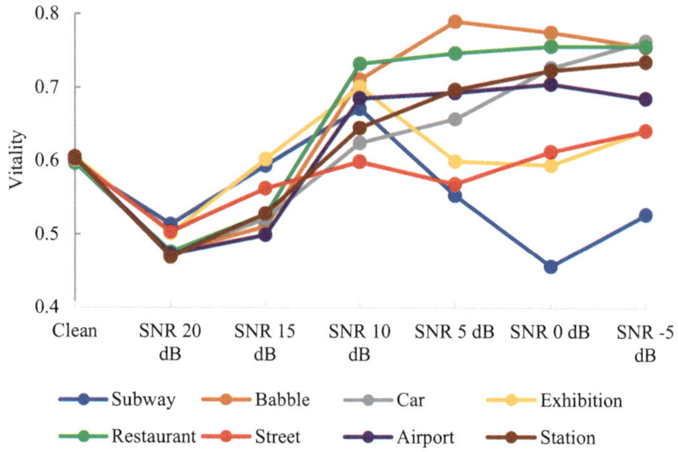

Fig. 4.5 Change in vitality due to noise. (Higuchi et al. 2018)

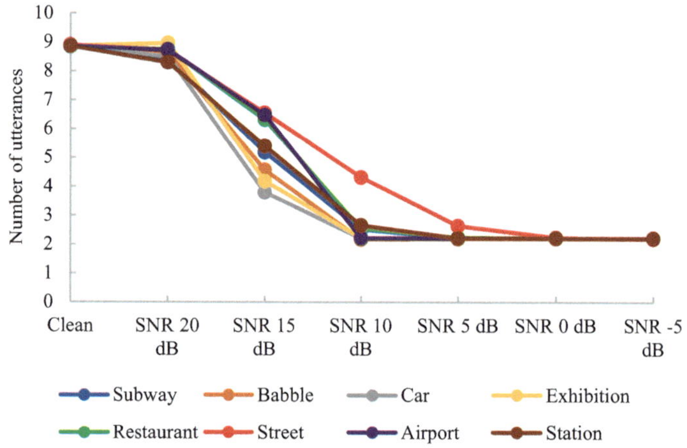

Fig. 4.6 Change in number of detected utterances. (Higuchi et al. 2018)

4.6 Multilingual Verification

The validation of MIMOSYS has mainly been conducted on Japanese speakers. However, ST, the basis of MIMOSYS, does not rely on a language model, but adopts acoustic features to estimate emotions, such that the algorithm can be applied to speakers of other languages without modification. Therefore, the University of Tokyo validated the performance of MIMOSYS across multiple languages using the MIMOSYS application for social implementation experiments.

MIMOSYS v2 for Android and iOS was released in April 2018 and at the end of January 2019, respectively. The analysis results of the data collected using

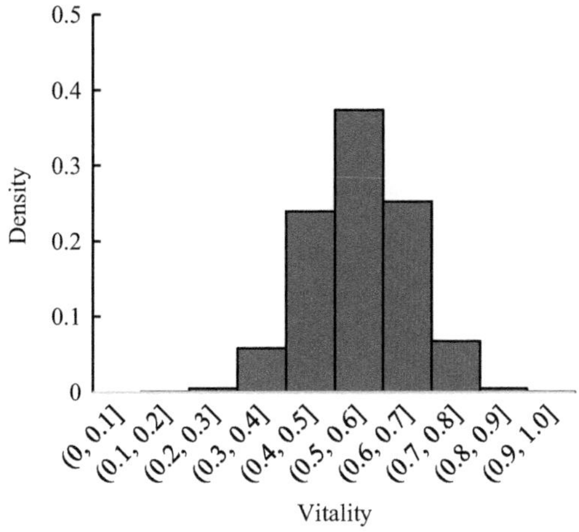

Fig. 4.7 Vitality distribution of Japanese speakers

MIMOSYS v2 are obtained. Figure 4.2 presents the distributions illustrated in Figs. 4.7 and 4.8 for Japanese speakers and speakers of other languages, respectively. A significant difference was identified between the distributions owing to the large sample size. However, because the effect size was negligible (−0.0007), we concluded that there was no difference in MIMOSYS between the cases of Japanese speakers and other language speakers.

4.7 Attempts to Improve Accuracy Using Statistical Inference Methods

MIMOSYS currently calculates mental activity based on the average and fluctuation of vitality over 2 weeks to monitor mental health. However, statistical inference methods can possibly estimate mental health by utilizing smaller amounts of data.

In this section, we focus on the fact that the distribution of vitality differs for each utterance and introduce a study that obtained the likelihood distribution for each utterance and adopted Bayesian inference to estimate mental states.

Bayes' theorem used in Bayesian inference is expressed by Eq. 4.1.

$$P(H|d) = \frac{P(d|H)}{P(d)} P(H) \tag{4.1}$$

Equation 4.1 states that the prior probability of a hypothesis is updated as the posterior probability after an event is observed. Considering this operation as a single step, Eq. 4.1 in step i can be expressed as follows:

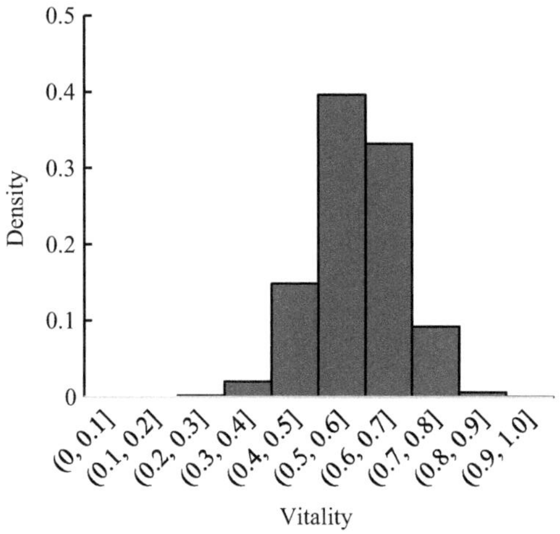

Fig. 4.8 Vitality distribution of non-Japanese speakers

$$P_{S(i+1)} = \frac{P_{sj}(v)}{P_{ij}(v)} P_{Si} \tag{4.2}$$

where P_S, P_{severe}, and P_{mild} represent the probability of major depressive disorder, severe probability, and mild probability, respectively. In addition, $P_{Sj(v)}$ denotes the probability density distribution of the vitality v of utterance number j in the severe or mild state. The probability density distribution of vitality is assumed to be a normal distribution and is expressed as Eq. 4.3 using the mean and standard deviation for state S and utterance number j. Furthermore, $P_{ij}(v)$ represents the probability density distribution of vitality v at step i and utterance number j.

$$P_{Sj}(v) = \frac{1}{\sqrt{2\pi\sigma^2}} \exp\left(-\frac{\left(v - \mu_{Sj}\right)^2}{\sigma_{Sj}^2} \right) \tag{4.3}$$

$P_{ij}(v)$ is the distribution of the occurrence probability of vitality v and is calculated as in Eq. 4.4 using the prior probability.

$$P_{ij}(v) = P_{\text{severe}i} P_{\text{severe}j}(v) + P_{\text{mild}i} P_{\text{mild}j}(v) \tag{4.4}$$

In the initial state before vitality v is observed, the mild and severe states are considered to have equal probabilities, and the equation is set as Equation 4.5.

$$P_{\text{severe}0} = P_{\text{mild}0} = 0.5 \tag{4.5}$$

Subsequently, each time vitality v is observed from an utterance, the probabilities of minor and severe cases are calculated based on Eq. 4.3, the occurrence probability of vitality is calculated from Eq. 4.4, and the posterior probability after observing vitality is calculated using Eq. 4.2. This operation was performed from speech

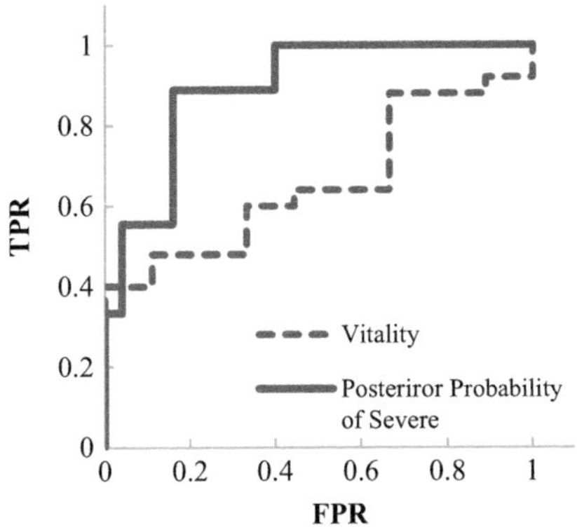

Fig. 4.9 ROC curve for separate severely depressed patient by posterior probability using Bayesian inference

number $j = 1$ to 20, and the severity probability P_{severe20} was adopted as an indicator of mental state estimation.

Figure 4.9 presents the receiver operating characteristic (ROC) curve for P_{severe20},which indicates the ability to distinguish between mild and severe patients. As illustrated in Fig. 4.9, the likelihood distribution $P_{\text{severe}j}(v)$ has the ability to separate mild and severe states better than the conventional method, which takes the average of each utterance.

This result suggests that a combination of $P_{\text{severe}i}$ and statistical methods can be expected to provide more accurate results than the estimation of severity using $P_{\text{severe}i}$ alone. MIMOSYS is expected to expand its range of applications because the likelihood distributions for all groups of states are known.

4.8 Conclusion

In this section, we discussed the results obtained from the validation of MIMOSYS to expand its range of applications. Section 4.2 demonstrated that differences in sex and age exhibited no effect. Section 4.3 verified that spontaneous speech outputs higher values than fixed-phrase speech. Section 4.4 demonstrated that the effect of the audio format exhibited a high correlation between the output of speech downsampled to 8 kHz and that of the original format. Section 4.5, which presented the effects of the noise environment, verified that MIMOSYS is affected by noise and that appropriate noise reduction measures are necessary. Section 4.6 demonstrated that MIMOSYS is not affected by language. In Sect. 4.7, the attempts to improve accuracy via statistical inference methods verified that Bayesian inference could be applied to further improve accuracy. We expect that the findings of this study will guide the development of novel products using MIMOSYS.

References

Hagiwara N, Omiya Y, Shinohara S, Nakamura M, Higuchi M, Mitsuyoshi S, Tokuno S (2017). Difference in voice analysis result by pre-and post-processing of telephone line. In: 2017 39th annual international conference of the IEEE engineering in medicine and biology society (EMBC). IEEE, Jeju, pp 242–245

Higuchi M, Shinohara S, Nakamura M, Omiya Y, Hagiwara N, Takano T, Mitsuyoshi S, Tokuno S (2018) Accuracy evaluation for mental health indicator based on vocal analysis in noisy environments. J Inf Commun Eng 4(1):217–222

Chapter 5
Stress and Depressive Symptoms: Validation of MIMOSYS (Clinical)

Masakazu Higuchi

5.1 Introduction

In the development of the mind monitoring system (MIMOSYS), the number of participants involved in the voice used to create the algorithm was insufficient (Shinohara et al. 2021). In addition, because the voice patterns and recording locations of healthy individuals and patients were different, the performance of the algorithm must be examined in various environments.

Therefore, to verify the performance of the algorithm, we collected voice recordings in various clinical settings and analyzed the voices using MIMOSYS.

5.2 MIMOSYS Analysis of Healthy Individuals and Depressed Patients

First, we collected voice recordings of healthy individuals and patients with depression and analyzed them using MIMOSYS (Tokuno 2016a).

Figure 5.1 shows the vitality of MIMOSYS for 26 healthy individuals and 8 patients. The vertical columns of the graph represent values measured multiple times for the same person. As can be seen, the vitalities in the healthy group widely fluctuated on a daily basis, whereas those of the patient group were

M. Higuchi (✉)
Department of Bioengineering, Graduate School of Engineering, The University of Tokyo, Bunkyo-ku, Tokyo, Japan
e-mail: higuchi@bioeng.t.u-tokyo.ac.jp

S. Tokuno, H. Nakamura (eds.), *Voice Biomarkers*,
https://doi.org/10.1007/978-981-96-3109-4_5

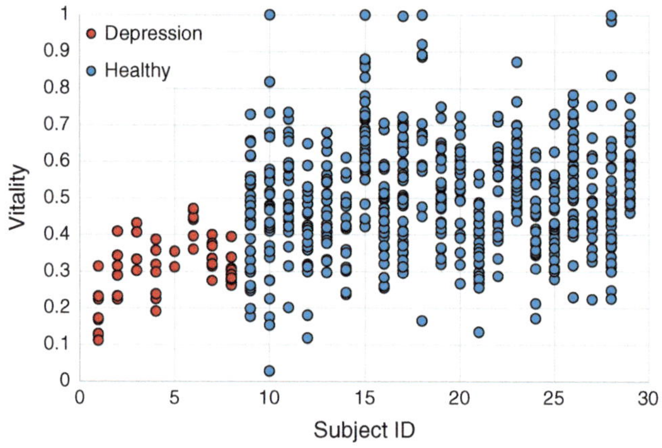

Fig. 5.1 Vitality distribution of the healthy and patient groups. (Modified from Tokuno 2016a)

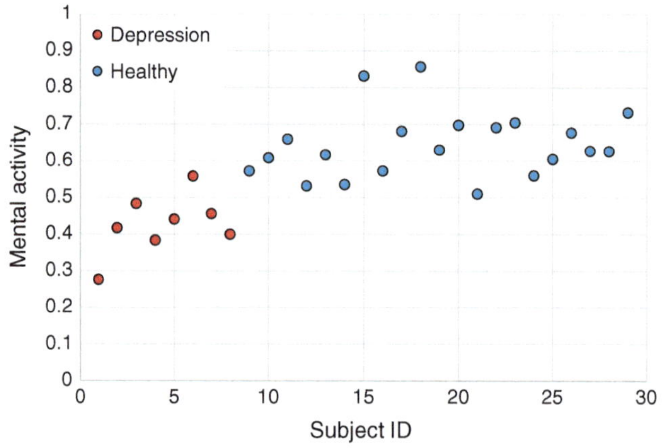

Fig. 5.2 Mental activity distribution of the healthy and patient groups. (Modified from Tokuno 2016a)

distributed in a lower area with less fluctuations. Low values of the healthy group from those of the patient group could be barely distinguished using vitality. Figure 5.2 shows the mental activity of MIMOSYS for the subject groups. Mental activity is an index that considers the mean and variance of vitality under the assumption that the differences in the mean and variance of vitality between the healthy and patient groups properly represent the differences between these groups; thus, the two groups were divided with a sufficient discriminative power, as assumed.

5.3 Relationship Between the MIMOSYS, Biological, and Questionnaire Indicators

Depressed and stressed individuals have decreased levels of brain-derived neurotrophic factor (BDNF) and increased levels of interleukin-1 receptor antagonist (IL-1ra) in their blood (Suzuki et al. 2014; Maes et al. 1995). The General Health Questionnaire 30 (GHQ30) (Goldberg 1978) is a self-administered questionnaire widely used to diagnose depression, similar to the Beck Depression Inventory (BDI) (Beck et al. 1961). We examined the relationship between these measures and the vitality of MIMOSYS (Shinohara et al. 2017; Nakamura et al. 2019).

The participants were 32 members of the Japan Self-Defense Forces Airborne Brigade during ranger training under an extreme stress. The training took place over a 9-week period. Blood samples, voice recordings, and self-administered questionnaires were obtained before, during (3 weeks after the start of training), and after (3–5 days after the end of training) the ranger training. Voice was recorded using an MS-PST1 medical recorder (Noritsu Koki, Japan) equipped with an AT9944 directional microphone (Audio-Technica, Japan).

Figure 5.3 shows the values of (a) the self-administered questionnaire GHQ30, (b) blood index BDNF, and (c) vitality before, during, and after the ranger training. In each sub-figure, the data before, during, and after training are shown from left to right. Higher scores of GHQ30 and lower scores of BDNF indicate higher levels of stress and depression. Each index showed a similar trend with the highest stress level during the training.

Figure 5.4 shows the values of (a) the blood index IL-1ra and (b) vitality before, during, and after the ranger training. The IL-1ra and vitality evaluations exhibited symmetrical temporal changes in the stress level, suggesting a physiological basis for the stress evaluation using vitality.

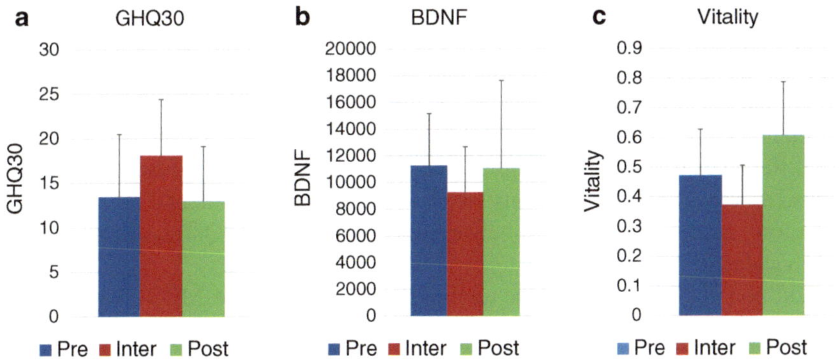

Fig. 5.3 GHQ30, BDNF, and vitality averages before, during, and after the ranger training. (Modified from Shinohara et al. 2017)

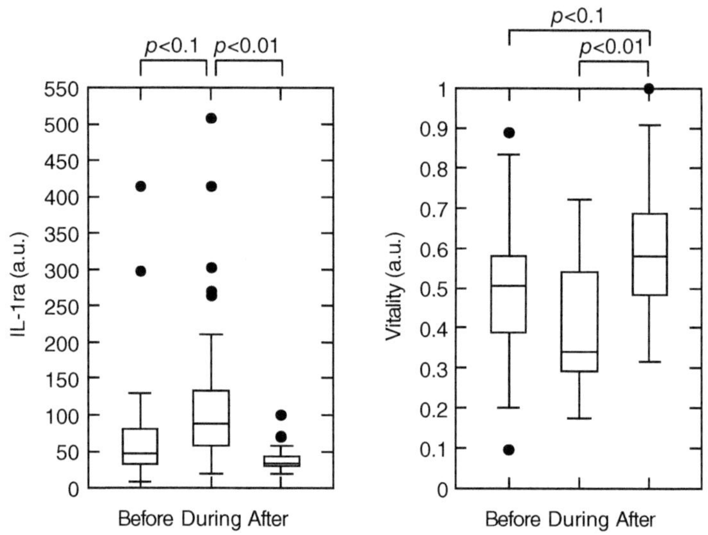

Fig. 5.4 Distributions of IL-1ra and vitality before, during, and after the ranger training

In addition, with the cooperation of a company, we assessed the mental health status of approximately 50 truck drivers using voice recordings immediately before and after work (Shinohara et al. 2015).

In this study, GHQ30 was evaluated once at the beginning of the experimental period followed by a second evaluation approximately 80 days after the first evaluation. Subsequently, the vitality index was calculated for each voice data for a total of 2 weeks, 1 week before, and after each GHQ30 test; the vitality average was used as the voice index at the time of each GHQ30 test. The voices of the dialogue between the subjects and manager were recorded using a PM-240 hand microphone (TOA, Kobe, Japan).

The results of the analysis revealed a negative correlation between the difference in the first and second scores of the GHQ30 items that were "general illness tendency," "physical symptoms," "suicidal ideation and depression tendency," and "total" and the difference between the first and second vitalities. Table 5.1 shows the correlation coefficients between the differences in the scores for each GHQ30 item and differences in vitalities. A higher GHQ30 score indicates a worse mental health status, whereas a higher vitality represents a healthier mental health status. Therefore, negative correlations between changes in the GHQ30 score and vitality were validated.

Additionally, we examined the relationship between the MIMOSYS vitality and Hamilton depression rating scale (HDRS) (Hamilton 1960) in patients with a major depressive disorder (Higuchi et al. 2018).

In this study, voices of patients undergoing treatments for major depressive disorders at a hospital were recorded. Thirty patients (19 men and 11 women) were included in the study. Voices were recorded in a hospital examination room, and

Table 5.1 Correlation coefficients between the GHQ30 item score and vitality differences ($*p < 0.1$, $**p < 0.05$, $***p < 0.01$)

GHQ30 item	Correlation coefficient
General illness tendency	−0.547***
Physical symptoms	−0.367*
Sleep disorder	0.016
Social activity disorder	−0.281
Anxiety and dysthymia	−0.004
Suicidal ideation and depression tendency	−0.416**
Total	−0.468**

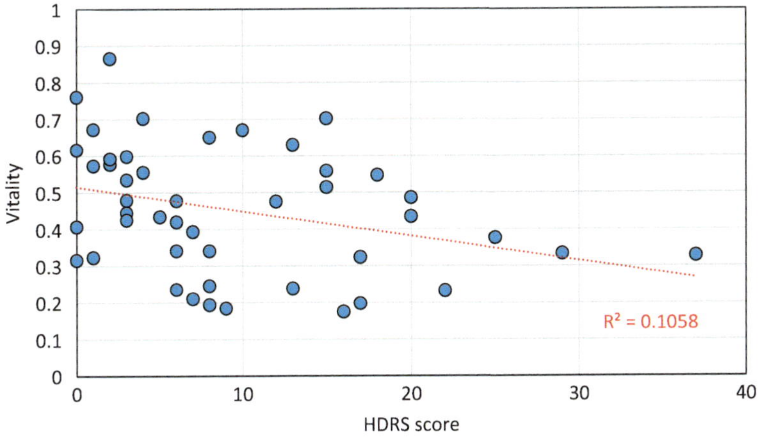

Fig. 5.5 Scatterplot of the vitality index and HDRS scores

patients were requested to read fixed Japanese phrases. A portable recorder R-26 (Roland, Japan) was used for voice recording. Because some patients were examined multiple times and voices were recorded each time, a total of 46 voice data points were collected (34 males and 12 females). A 21-item version of HDRS was administered by a physician to assess the severity of the depression.

A scatterplot of vitality and HDRS scores is shown in Fig. 5.5. The correlation coefficient between the vitality and HDRS score was −0.33, which was considerable at a significance level of 5%, indicating a weak negative correlation. Therefore, patients with more severe depression tend to have a lower vitality.

Subsequently, we evaluated the discriminative performance of the two groups of patients using the vitality index. The HDRS score of the healthy group was less than 5 points, whereas that of the depressed group was 5 points or higher. The HDRS cutoff point was determined according to the evaluation criteria for the 21-item version of HDRS proposed by the Japan Committee for Prevention and Treatment of Depression (Japan Committee for Prevention and Treatment of Depression 2010). Figure 5.6 shows the distribution of vitality for the two groups. The t-test results for

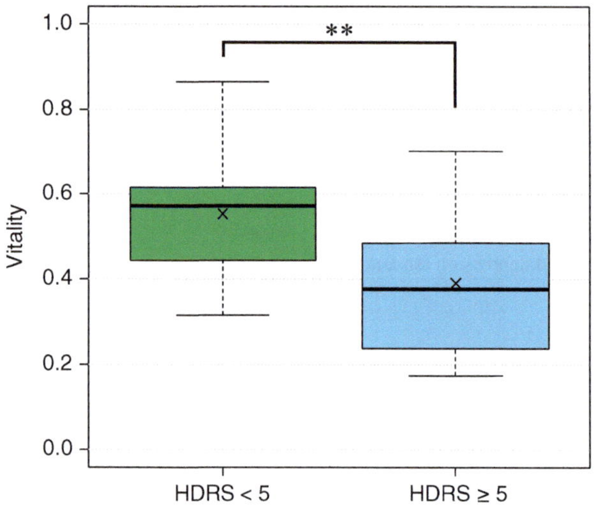

Fig. 5.6 Vitality distribution of healthy and depressed groups ($* * p < 0.01$)

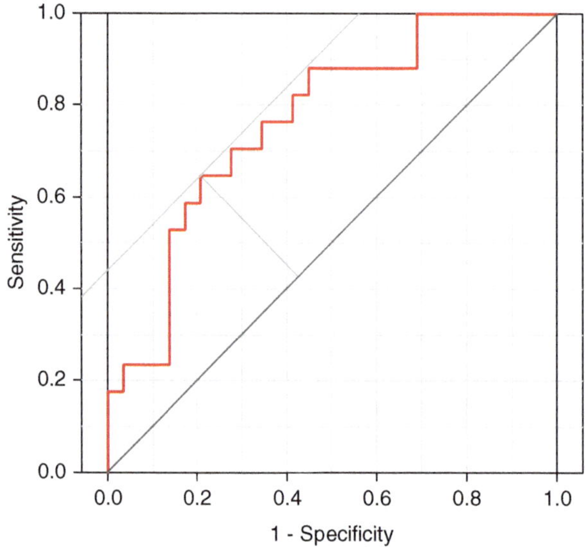

Fig. 5.7 ROC curve for discriminative evaluation of normal and depressed groups using vitality

the mean vitality values for the two groups exhibited a considerable difference at a significance level of 1%. Figure 5.7 shows the receiver operating characteristic (ROC) curve, which represents the discriminant performance of the two groups using vitality. The area under the curve (AUC) for the ROC curve was 0.77, and the sensitivity and specificity at the best cutoff point were 0.65 and 0.79, respectively.

The subjects in the healthy group were considered to be in remission after treatment. In addition, the results confirmed that vitality can slightly distinguish healthy individuals from patients with depression.

5.4 Validation of MIMOSYS on Smartphones

5.4.1 Implementation of MIMOSYS on Smartphones

Easy application of MIMOSYS in clinical practices is desirable. As the performance of mobile device platforms has significantly improved, smartphones can perform a moderate level of computational processing. In addition, smartphones are widely used as they are indispensable in our daily lives; thus, they are appropriate tools for continuous and noninvasive monitoring of users' biometrics and other health information. Many studies have been conducted on the development of mental health applications for mobile devices and detection of stress using smartphones (Lu et al. 2012; Donker et al. 2013).

We implemented MIMOSYS on a smartphone with a concentration on the voices of phone calls in our daily lives (Tokuno 2015, 2016b, 2019a, b, c, 2020a). Therefore, the mental health could be readily monitored on a daily basis while preventing mental disorders, such as depression.

5.4.2 Validation of the MIMOSYS Smartphone Application

By implementing MIMOSYS on smartphones, various voices can be readily analyzed. We rented smartphones with installed MIMOSYS application to 50 subjects (39 males and 11 females) and collected and analyzed voice data for approximately 2 months (Shinohara et al. 2017; Hagiwara et al. 2017). The subjects were requested to make daily recordings by reading fixed Japanese phrases. In total, 4357 fixed Japanese phrase recordings were obtained. The MIMOSYS application deleted voice recordings after the analysis; however, the results and user information were aggregated and stored in a database via Wi-Fi. The analysis results were retrieved from the database. In addition, a BDI test was conducted at the beginning of voice acquisition.

First, the relationship between the MIMOSYS and BDI test scores was examined using only the voice data from 2 weeks after the BDI test was conducted, because BDI test scores may change over a medium to long term. The mental activity, which is a mid- to long-term index, was calculated based on the vitality calculated from the 2-week voice data and used as the mental activity index at the time the BDI test was conducted. The correlations between the BDI scores and vitality and BDI scores and mental activity are shown in Figs. 5.8 and 5.9, respectively. The correlation

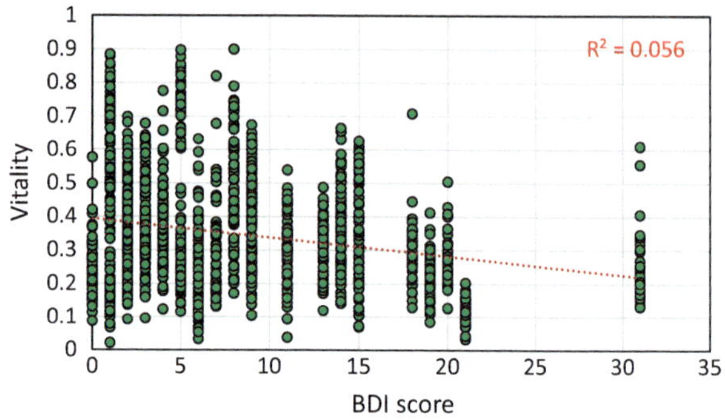

Fig. 5.8 Scatterplot between the vitality and BDI score. (Modified from Hagiwara et al. 2017)

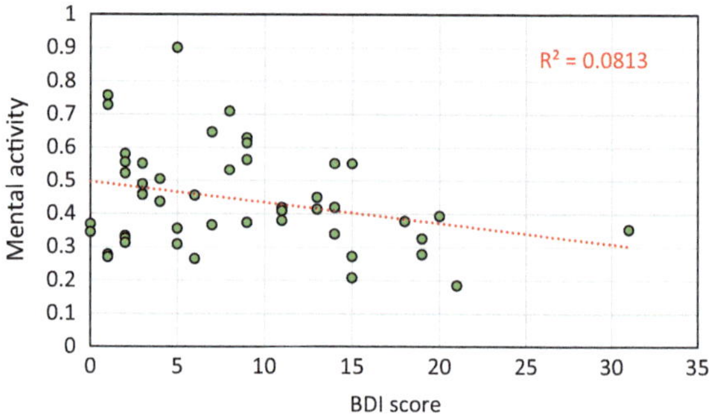

Fig. 5.9 Scatterplot between the mental activity and BDI score. (Modified from Hagiwara et al. 2017)

coefficients of the BDI score with vitality and mental activity were −0.237 and −0.285, respectively. A higher BDI score indicates a worse mental health status, whereas a higher vitality represents a healthier mental health status. Therefore, negative correlations between BDI and the two indices of MIMOSYS were validated by these results.

Subsequently, we evaluated the performance of MIMOSYS in distinguishing subjects who were considered to have a poor mental health by voice. According to the BDI evaluation criteria (Beck et al. 1988), subjects were divided into two groups: a low-risk disease group with a BDI score of 18 or less and a high-risk disease group with a BDI score greater than 18. There were 43 subjects in the low-risk disease group and 5 in the high-risk disease group. Figures 5.10 and 5.11 show the distribution of vitality and mental activity of the two groups, respectively. The t-test results revealed that the vitality and mental activity indices of the two groups were significantly different. Figures 5.12 and 5.13 show the ROC curves of the vitality and mental activity indices. Moreover, the sensitivity and specificity at each best cutoff point are shown in Table 5.2. Moreover, AUCs of ROC for both the vitality and mental activity indices were approximately 0.8, indicating a reasonable discriminative performance.

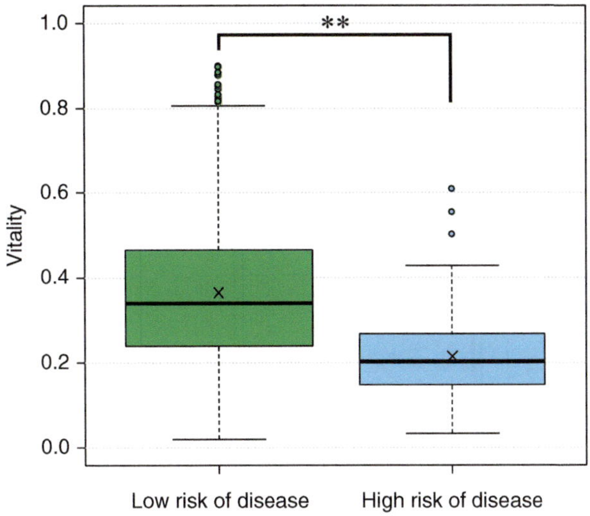

Fig. 5.10 Vitality distributions of low-risk and high-risk disease groups ($**p < 0.01$). (Modified from Hagiwara et al. 2017)

Fig. 5.11 Mental activity distributions of low-risk and high-risk disease groups ($**p < 0.01$). (Modified from Hagiwara et al. 2017)

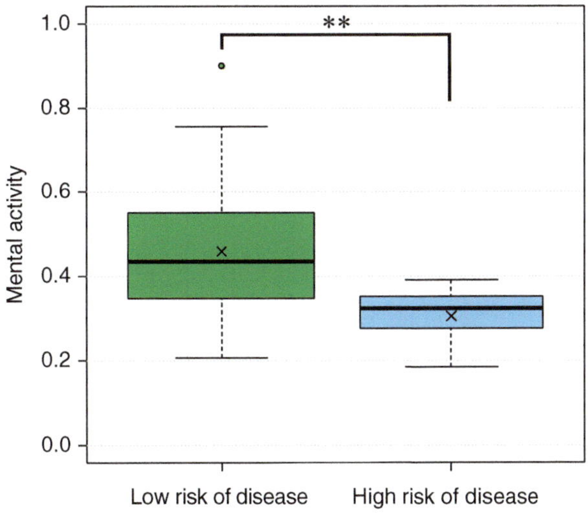

5.4.3 Large-Scale Social Implementation Targeting an Unspecified Number of Smartphone Users

We made the MIMOSYS smartphone application available to the public for a prospective study and acquired MIMOSYS data from an unspecified number of smartphone users who agreed to participate in the study over a 2-year period. Subsequently,

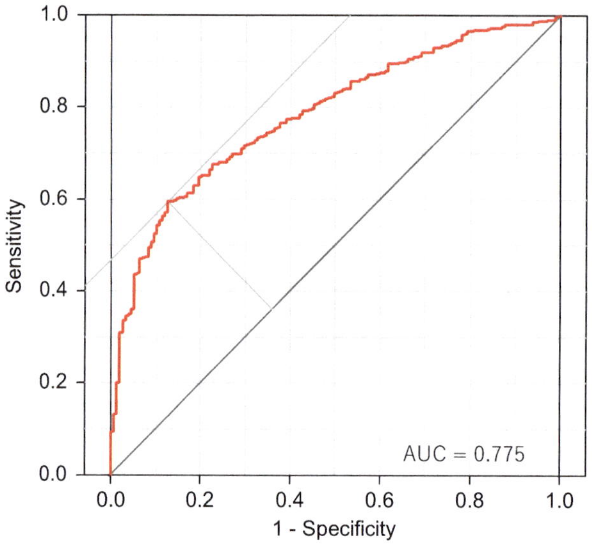

Fig. 5.12 ROC for discriminative evaluation of low-risk and high-risk disease groups using vitality. (Modified from Hagiwara et al. 2017)

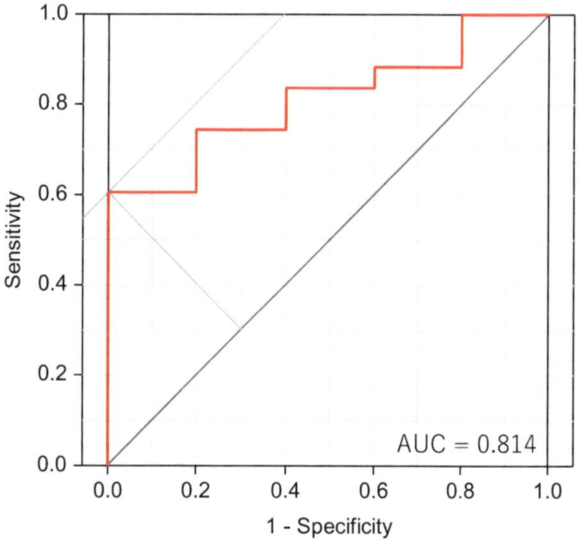

Fig. 5.13 ROC for discriminative evaluation of low-risk and high-risk disease groups using mental activity. (Modified from Hagiwara et al. 2017)

we verified the characteristics and effectiveness of MIMOSYS from various perspectives using acquired data (Higuchi et al. 2020).

When MIMOSYS was installed on a smartphone, consent for participation in the study was requested at the time of initial use, and attribute data, such as sex, age, medical history, current medical history, and place of residence, were obtained for

Table 5.2 Performance of MIMOSYS in discriminating low-risk and high-risk disease groups

Index	Sensitivity	Specificity
Vitality	0.80	0.64
Mental activity	1.0	0.61

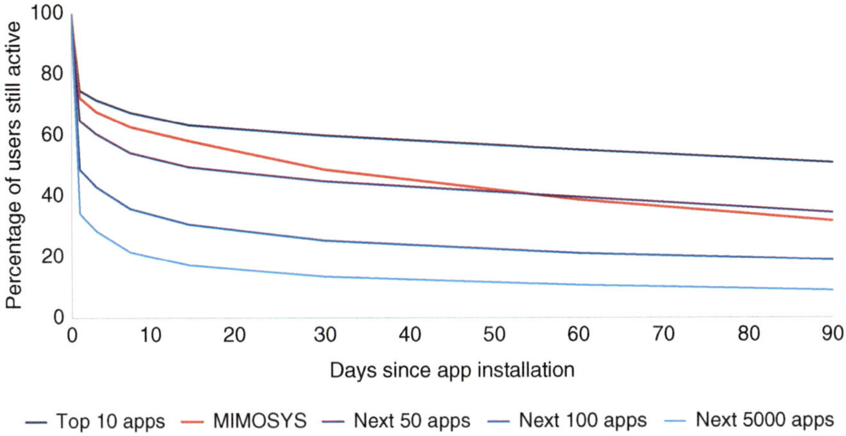

Fig. 5.14 Continuous usage rate for MIMOSYS and other smartphone applications. (Cited from Higuchi et al. 2020)

users who consented to participate in the study. In addition, the BDI test was conducted on the screen. Calls were privately made by the users themselves and conducted irregularly on their own smartphones. The application was downloaded approximately 3800 times during the data collection period, and the number of users who consented to participate in the study and analyzed at least one call using MIMOSYS was 1814. From these users, we obtained 183,490 data for effective vitality and 167,610 data for effective mental activity.

Continuous usage curves for MIMSYS and other smartphone applications are shown in Fig. 5.14. The continuous usage rate of MIMOSYS was comparable to that of the top 60 applications in the Google Play ranking. Because MIMOSYS automatically begins processing when a call is made, the user can use MIMOSYS without being aware of it; thus, MIMOSYS could maintain such a high continuous usage rate for an approximately long time. The monitoring system was designed to be used over a long period of time, and the automatic analysis of MIMOSYS calls was considered effective.

The distributions of the vitality and mental activity indices are shown in Figs. 5.15 and 5.16, respectively. According to the effect size in the goodness-of-fit test, the vitality and mental activity indices are normally distributed. Most parametric statistical analyses assume that the data under analysis follow a normal distribution; thus, the normal distribution of the obtained data is of great significance in subsequent statistical tests. Consequently, the vitality and mental activity indices were considered advantageous for statistical analysis.

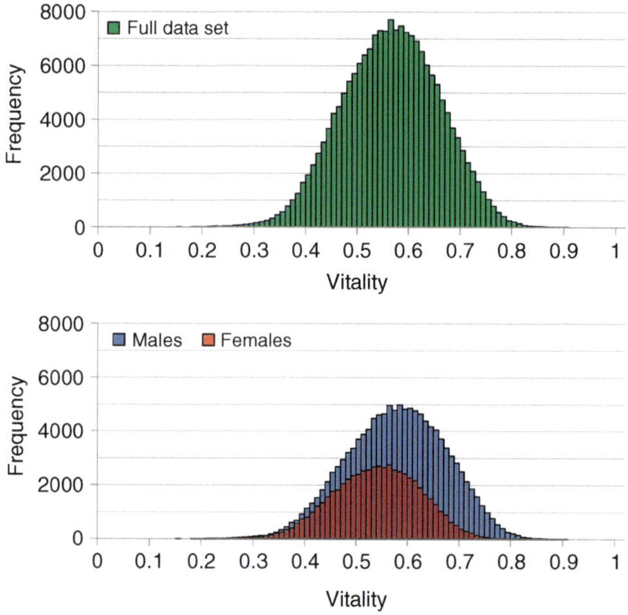

Fig. 5.15 Vitality distributions for the full set and by gender. (Cited from Higuchi et al. 2020)

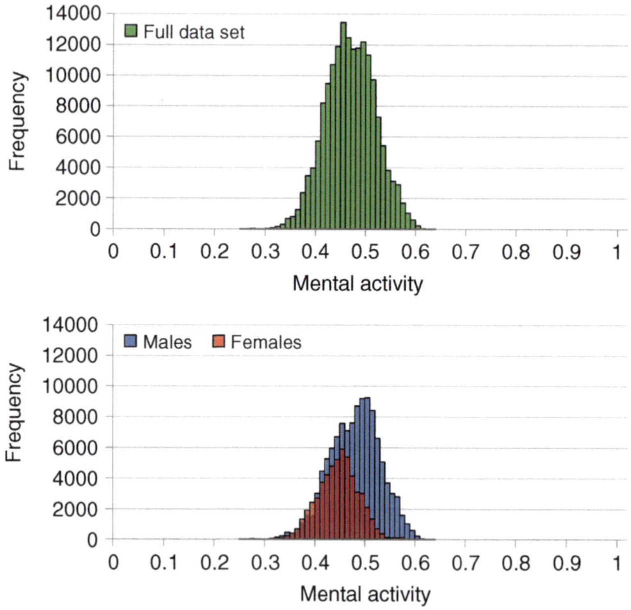

Fig. 5.16 Mental activity distributions for the full set and by gender. (Cited from Higuchi et al. 2020)

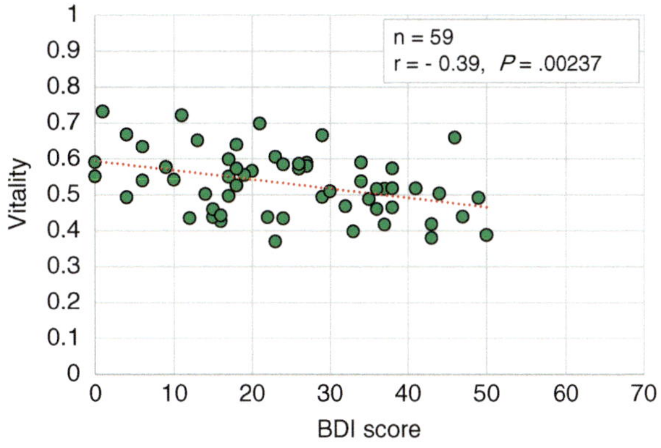

Fig. 5.17 Scatterplot of the BDI score and vitality index for users with depression. (Modified from Higuchi et al. 2020)

The vitality and mental activity indices tended to be lower for women than that of men. The prevalence of depression in women is higher than that in men (Weissman and Klerman 1977), and MIMOSYS may have detected this difference. In the data of users who were considered normal based on the BDI score, the effect size of the mean vitality in men and women was comparable. In contrast, the difference between the effect size of the mean vitality in men and women was not negligible in the data of users who could not be considered.

Figure 5.17 shows the correlation between the BDI score and vitality index of the users. Users were selected from those who were expected to seriously respond to the BDI test and reported depression in their current medical history. The first vitality measurement after the BDI test was selected and used in the analysis. We found a significant weak negative correlation between the BDI score and vitality index. Moreover, no significant correlation was found between the BDI score and latest mental activity within 2 weeks after the BDI test.

5.4.4 *Monitoring the Mental Health Status of Company's Employees*

Stress checks have recently become mandatory in Japan for business establishments with 50 employees or more. The purpose of this initiative is to prevent the occurrence of mental health problems by applying primary preventive measures to proactively avoid mental health problems and provide healthier workplace environments. In cooperation with a Japanese company, we monitored the mental health of employees using MIMOSYS (Tokuno 2020b).

Figure 5.18 shows an example of the monitoring results of the mental activity index of an employee of a company using the MIMOSYS smartphone application. Employees' mental activity began to drop at a certain point in time and remained low for a certain period of time. When an interview with an industrial physician was recommended close to the time of the lowest mental activity, the mental activity

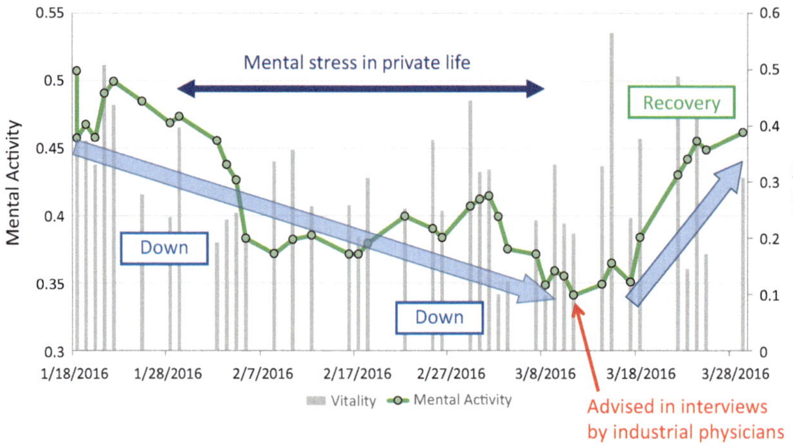

Fig. 5.18 Changes in mental activity for an employee of a company

exhibited a recovery trend. The results of the follow-up questionnaire revealed that the employee had been experiencing private problems during the period when the mental activity index was on a downward trend. Thus, MIMOSYS was effective as both a screening tool and monitoring tool.

5.5 Validation of the Number of Utterances in the MIMOSYS Analysis

MIMOSYS was developed to use voices of daily telephone calls. Because various utterances are included in natural speeches, such as telephone calls, the vitality index is calculated for each utterance and averaged and used as the final vitality index for the input voice. If a telephone call is difficult to use, it can be handled by inputting various fixed phrases as pseudo-calls. Therefore, a certain number of utterances is required to obtain stable results. In addition, six or more utterances should be empirically included in the speech to obtain a sufficient accuracy with MIMOSYS. However, when MIMOSYS is used for continuous monitoring of stress in members of various companies, less input utterances are desirable in daily measurements as it is an extremely key factor.

Research on mood often artificially induces participants to hold a specific mood, where verbal instruction is an induction method. In this method, participants are requested to read positive sentences to induce a pleasant mood and negative sentences to induce an unpleasant mood (Fiedler 2001); thus, readers' mood changes depending on the meaning of the sentences read. Because depressed people do not tend to express their emotions and their mood is not likely to change, the vitality index of depressed people is expected to differ from that of the healthy people when MIMOSYS is applied to utterances that induce pleasant/unpleasant emotions. If a characteristic trend in the difference is found, it may lead to a reduction in the number of input utterances.

Therefore, to achieve an accurate estimation of depression with a small number of input utterances, we evaluated the performance of MIMOSYS on the number of input utterances considering the semantic differences of utterances in self-reported healthy individuals and patients diagnosed with depression by a physician (Higuchi et al. 2022).

In this study, 130 subjects were recruited, including 93 patients undergoing treatment for major depressive disorder at a hospital and 37 self-reported healthy individuals. The severity of depression was evaluated by a physician using HDRS. According to the evaluation criteria for the 21-item HDRS (Japan Committee for Prevention and Treatment of Depression 2010), HDRS scores of less than 5 points were regarded as healthy subjects. Therefore, 92 and 38 participants were in the healthy and depressed groups, respectively. Voices were recorded in a hospital examination room using a portable recorder R-26 (Roland, Japan), and participants were requested to read 17 fixed Japanese phrases. Eleven fixed phrases did not contain emotions, where four and two fixed phrases contained positive and negative emotions, respectively. To maintain the number of positive, negative, and nonemotional phrases as equal as possible, four other phrases were selected. Therefore, ten phrases were used in the analysis. In this study, each phrase read by the subjects was considered to be one utterance, and all vitality indices in each phrase were averaged to form a standard vitality for each subject.

The results of this analysis are shown in Fig. 5.19. The green line represents AUC for the ROC curve obtained when the depression group was discriminated by the standard vitality. For each number of utterances, the red dots represent the largest AUC among AUCs for the ROC curves obtained when the depression group was discriminated by the vitality index calculated from the combined utterances, and the blue dots represent the smallest AUC. The black dots represent the mean AUC, where the upper and lower bars represent the standard error. The maximum AUC tended to increase when the number of utterances was small, reached the maximum value when the number of utterances was four, achieved a value larger than AUC by the standard vitality, and then decreased. The combination of utterances that yielded the maximum AUC tended to include more positive than negative utterances. However, the combination of utterances that yielded the minimum AUC tended to include more negative than positive utterances, because the reader's mood changed depending on the meaning of the utterance. That is, the healthy group tended to feel more energetic when positive utterances were read because of their rich emotional expressions, whereas the depressed group tended to feel less energetic even when positive utterances were read because of their poor emotional expressions. Therefore, it was thought that reading many positive utterances increases the difference between the vitality indices of the healthy and depressed groups. However, when negative utterances were read, the healthy group became depressed and lost energy, and their energy level became the same as that of the depressed group, while the depressed group did not change their mood; thus, the difference in vitality between the two groups was small. Consequently, depressive states could be estimated with

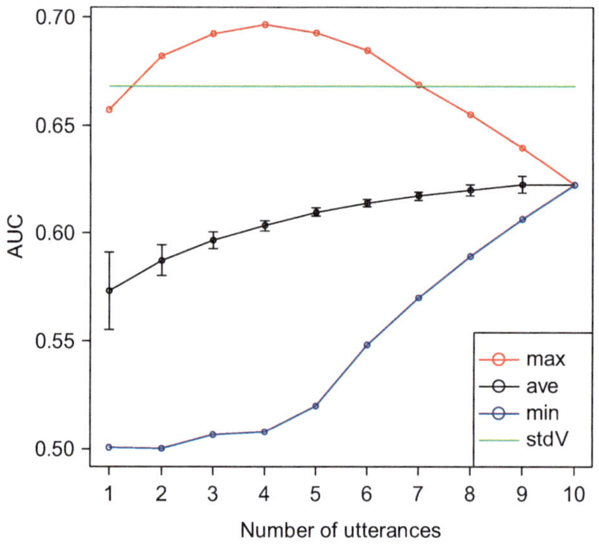

Fig. 5.19 Discrimination accuracy between the healthy and depressed groups with respect to number of utterances. (Cited from Higuchi et al. 2022)

a sufficient accuracy using MIMOSYS and the lowest number of utterances when three to four positive utterances were included.

5.6 Multilingual Validation of MIMOSYS

MIMOSYS was developed using the Japanese voice. Thus, we decided to examine its performance in languages other than Japanese (Popa et al. 2019; Uraguchi et al. 2018).

Popa et al. collected data on a daily basis using the MIMOSYS smartphone application with 20 students at Transylvania University in Brasov, Romania (Popa et al. 2019). The results of the data analysis showed that a slight correlation between the emotional components of the voice existed; thus, MIMOSYS might be potentially used for languages other than Japanese.

Uraguchi et al. conducted a voice analysis using MIMOSYS on Romanian and Russian native-speaking subjects (Uraguchi et al. 2018). Nineteen males (16 Romanian and 3 Russian) and 141 females (131 Romanian and 10 Russian) recorded fixed-phrase voices using a portable recorder R-26 (Roland, Japan). Voices were recorded twice at a 2-week interval. The BDI test was conducted simultaneously. In the voice analysis, subjects were divided into the low- and high-risk depression groups based on the BDI score with a threshold of 17 points. In addition, the discrimination performance of the two groups was evaluated using the vitality index. In addition, participants were divided into the low- and high-risk suicide groups

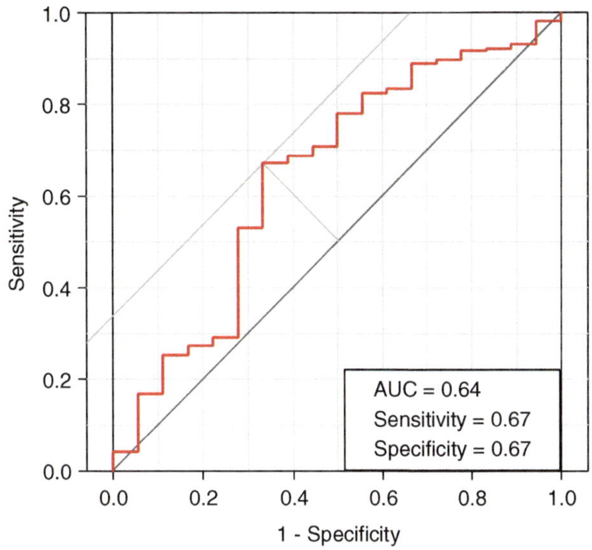

Fig. 5.20 ROC for the discriminant evaluation of low- and high risk depression groups using the vitality index

based on the score of question 9 (suicidal ideation) of the BDI test with a threshold of 2 points; the discrimination performance of the two groups was evaluated using the vitality index. Figures 5.20 and 5.21 show the discrimination performance of the low- and high-risk depression groups and low- and high-risk suicide groups, respectively, as evaluated using the ROC curves. The results suggest that the vitality index can discriminate between people with a strong suicidal ideation.

5.7 Conclusions

To validate the performance of MIMOSYS, we collected and analyzed voice recordings at various clinical settings.

The vitality and mental activity indices of patients with depression were clearly lower than those of healthy individuals. In addition, the stress evaluation using the vitality index revealed temporal changes corresponding to the stress evaluation by BDNF and IL-1ra, suggesting a physiological basis for the stress evaluation using the vitality index. Furthermore, vitality was correlated with typical depression evaluation indices, such as GHQ30, BDI, and HDRS, by self-administered questionnaires and physician interviews. In addition, the mental activity index was correlated with the BDI score. These results indicated the validity of measuring mental health by the vitality and mental activity indices.

We developed the MIMOSYS smartphone application and constructed an environment that enabled data acquisition from a wider cohort. The continuous usage

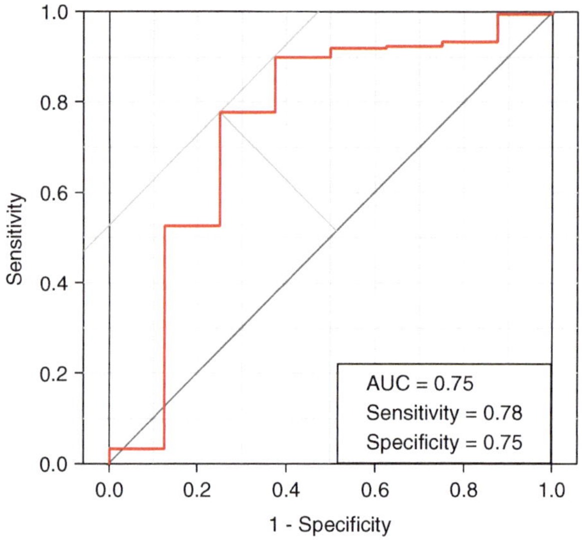

Fig. 5.21 ROC for the discriminant evaluation of low- and high risk suicide groups using the vitality index

rate of the MIMOSYS application was comparable to that of the top 60 applications in the Google Play ranking, demonstrating its effectiveness as a monitoring system. The statistical properties of the vitality and mental activity indices of several thousand users were obtained and analyzed. It was shown that the vitality and mental activity indices followed normal distributions, which is advantageous for a parametric statistical analysis. In addition, vitality and mental activity tended to be lower in females, which may have detected differences in depression rates between males and females. However, the label data from general users may not be sufficiently reliable, highlighting the issues of obtaining data from general users and limitations of conducting analysis using general data.

In addition, stress monitoring of company employees was conducted using the MIMOSYS application. We confirmed that some subjects exhibited changes in mental activity consistent with life events, indicating the possibility of early detection of excessive stress in work environments using MIMOSYS. Appropriate number of utterances to be input to MIMOSYS for continuous monitoring of stress in companies was examined with an aim to reduce required daily measurements. Therefore, depression could be estimated with a sufficient accuracy when three to four utterances contained positive meanings.

The effectiveness of MIMOSYS in Japan has been sufficiently validated. Because our voice technology is technically considered language-independent, we validated MIMOSYS overseas. Consequently, MIMOSYS could discriminate people with strong suicidal ideation using the vitality index of foreign people whose native language was either Romanian or Russian. Thus, MIMOSYS could effectively perform in two other languages; however, its performance in more languages will be investigated in future studies.

References

Beck AT, Ward CH, Mendelson M, Mock J, Erbaugh J (1961) An inventory for measuring depression. Arch Gen Psychiatry 4(6):561–571

Beck AT, Steer RA, Garbin MGJ (1988) Psychometric properties of the Beck depression inventory twenty-five years of evaluation. Clin Psych Rev 8:77–100

Donker T, Petrie K, Proudfoot J, Clarke J, Birch MR, Christensen H (2013) Smartphones for smarter delivery of mental health programs: a systematic review. J Med Internet Res 15(11):e247

Fiedler K (2001) Affective influences on social information processing. In: Forgas JP (ed) Handbook of affect and social cognition. Lawrence Erlbaum Associates Publishers, Hoboken, pp 163–185

Goldberg DP (1978) Manual of the general health questionnaire. NFER Publishing, Windsor

Hagiwara N, Omiya Y, Shinohara S, Nakamura M, Higuchi M, Mitsuyoshi S, Yasunaga H, Tokuno S (2017) Validity of mind monitoring system as a mental health indicator using voice. Adv Sci Technol Eng Syst J 2(3):338–344

Hamilton M (1960) A rating scale for depression. J Neurol Neurosurg Psychiatry 23:56–62

Higuchi M, Nakamura M, Shinohara S, Omiya Y, Hagiwara N, Takano T, Toda H, Saito T, Yoshino A, Mitsuyoshi S, Tokuno S (2018) Effectiveness of voice-based mental health evaluation indicator in estimating depression. In: Proceedings of symposium of human communication group (HCG Symposium 2018), Ise, 12–14 December 2018 (in Japanese)

Higuchi M, Nakamura M, Shinohara S, Omiya Y, Takano T, Mitsuyoshi S, Tokuno S (2020) Effectiveness of a voice-based mental health evaluation system for mobile devices: prospective study. JMIR Form Res 4(7):e16455

Higuchi M, Sonota N, Nakamura M, Miyazaki K, Shinohara S, Omiya Y, Takano T, Mitsuyoshi S, Tokuno S (2022) Performance evaluation of a voice-based depression assessment system considering the number and type of input utterances. Sensors 22(1):67

Japan Committee for Prevention and Treatment of Depression (2010) Key aspects of treatment of depression-10 [Translated from Japanese]. https://www.jcptd.jp/medical/point_10.pdf. Accessed 25 Mar 2022

Lu H, Rabbi M, Chittaranjan GT, Frauendorfer D, Mast MS, Campbell AT, Gatica-Perez D, Choudhury T (2012) Stresssense: detecting stress in unconstrained acoustic environments using smartphones. In: Proceedings of the 2012 ACM conference on Ubiquitous computing, Pittsburgh, 5–8 September 2012, pp 351–360

Maes M, Vandoolaeghe E, Ranjan R, Bosmans E, Bergmans R, Desnyder R (1995) Increased serum interleukin-1-receptor-antagonist concentrations in major depression. J Affect Disord 36:29–36

Nakamura M, Suzuki G, Shinohara S, Omiya Y, Higuchi M, Takano T, Mitsuyoshi S, Kobayashi N, Tokuno S (2019) Relation between stress estimated by voice analysis and blood interleukin-1 receptor antagonist in high-intensity training. In: Abstracts of the 41st international engineering in medicine and biology conference (EMBC 2019), Berlin, 23–27 July 2019

Popa D, Nechita F, Coman C, Barbu S, Shinohara S, Tokuno S, Nakamura M, Takano T (2019) Mind monitoring system (MIMOSYS) for mental and wellbeing of young students. In: Abstract of X Simpósio Nacional de Investigação em Psicologia, Madeira, 27–29 June 2019

Shinohara S, Nakamura M, Omiya Y, Takagi H, Ushiwatari A, Mitsuyoshi S, Tokuno S (2015) Validity of mental health check by voice compared to psychological test. In: Proceedings of symposium of human communication group (HCG Symposium 2015), Toyama, 16–18 December 2015 (in Japanese)

Shinohara S, Omiya Y, Hagiwara N, Nakamura M, Higuchi M, Kirita T, Takano T, Mitsuyoshi S, Tokuno S (2017) Case studies of utilization of the mind monitoring system (MIMOSYS) using voice and its future prospects. Econophys Sociophys Other Multidiscip Sci J 7(1):7–12

Shinohara S, Nakamura M, Omiya Y, Higuchi M, Hagiwara N, Mitsuyoshi S, Toda H, Saito T, Tanichi M, Yoshino A, Tokuno S (2021) Depressive mood assessment method based on emotion level derived from voice: comparison of voice features of individuals with major depressive disorders and healthy controls. Int J Environ Res Public Health 18(10):5435

Suzuki G, Tokuno S, Nibuya M, Ishida T, Yamamoto T, Mukai Y, Tsumatori G, Scott D, Shimizu K (2014) Decreased plasma brain-derived neurotrophic factor and vascular endothelial growth factor concentrations during military training. PLoS ONE 9(2):e89455

Tokuno S (2015) The latest stress check technology for nurses [Translated from Japanese]. Monthly Nurs 35(9):67–76. (in Japanese)

Tokuno S (2016a) Verbal analysis of pathophysiology [Translated from Japanese]. Cell 48(14):673–676. (in Japanese)

Tokuno S (2016b) Medical evidence of voice pathophysiology analysis technology. In: Abstract of joint symposium with IT companies of the 7th Asia Pacific regional conference of the International Association for Suicide Prevention, Tokyo, 18–21 May 2016

Tokuno S (2019a) Further developing voice analysis technology capable of detecting changes in vocal patterns which signal changes in stress levels and depressive symptoms. Impact 2019(6):43–45

Tokuno S (2019b) Healthcare early detection technology: Voice analysis technology. Open Access Govern 2019(10):58–59

Tokuno S (2019c) On mental monitoring using voice emotion recognition technology [Translated from Japanese]. In: Nature forum: mental health and data science, Tokyo, 24 October 2019 (in Japanese)

Tokuno S (2020a) "MIMOSYS", a smartphone application to visualize stress conditions [Translated from Japanese]. In: The 20th annual meeting of the Japanese Society of Anti-Aging Medicine, Virtual, 25–27 September 2020 (in Japanese)

Tokuno S (2020b) A mind monitoring system: voice analysis technology. Open Access Govern 2020(1):196–197

Uraguchi T, Shinohara S, Negrea D, Ţaicu M, Săvoiu G, Omiya Y, Nakamura M, Higuchi M, Takano T, Hagiwara N, Mitsuyoshi S, Tokuno S (2018) Evaluation of mind monitoring system (MIMOSYS) by subjects with Romanian and Russian as their native language. In: Abstracts of the 40th international engineering in medicine and biology conference (EMBC 2018), Hawaii, 17–21 July 2018

Weissman MM, Klerman GL (1977) Sex differences and the epidemiology of depression. Arch Gen Psychiatry 34(1):98–111

Chapter 6
Stress and Depressive Symptoms: Utilization of MIMOSYS

Yasuhiro Omiya

6.1 Introduction

MIMOSYS has been validated in various fields, including validation in engineering and medicine, and has been used in various situations. In this section, case studies of individuals, collective cases such as institutions and companies, and examples of data collected through large-scale social implementation studies in relation to events are introduced.

6.2 Case Study of Monitoring the Mental State of an Individual

Tokuno reported the relationship between events that occurred around a woman and the results of a MIMOSYS analysis (Tokuno 2020a, b). The woman was 50 years old at the time and lived with her husband and three sons. Her eldest son was already independent, and her mother fought her illness in a remote area. The results of all her voice calls from August 2015 to March 2019 were analyzed using the MIMOSYS app and the relationship between various events.

Figure 6.1 shows trends in the woman's vitality and mental activities. The vitality index fluctuates greatly depending on the content of the conversation during the call and depending on the caller, while mental activity shows a trend over the past 2 weeks, including the time of the call. Changes in mental activity shown in orange indicate the woman's intensity of stress and depression.

Y. Omiya (✉)
Research and Development Department, PST Inc., Yokohama, Kanagawa, Japan
e-mail: omiya@medical-pst.com

S. Tokuno, H. Nakamura (eds.), *Voice Biomarkers*,
https://doi.org/10.1007/978-981-96-3109-4_6

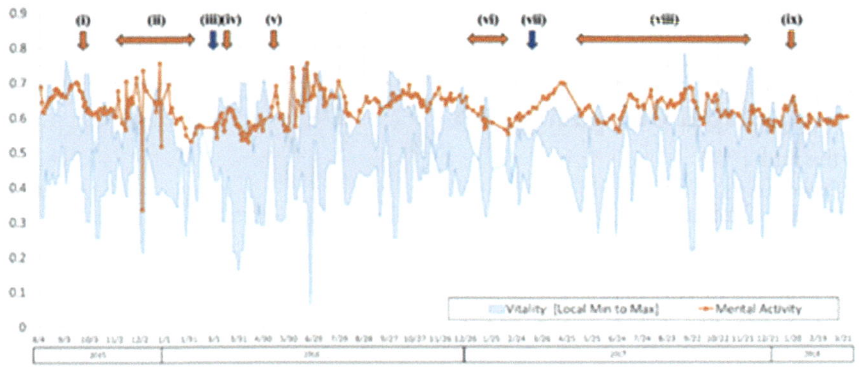

Fig. 6.1 Changes in the woman's vitality and mental activity

A discussion of the relationship between each event that occurred around him or her and the results analyzed using the MIMOSYS application is presented below.

(i) Her mother's death was a major event for her, and her vitality obviously decreased when she heard news of her mother's death.
(ii) Her two sons embarked on entrance examinations, and stress and fatigue caused a brief and rapid fluctuation in her mental activity, which subsequently decreased.
(iii) She started to recover upon hearing that her third son had passed his examination.
(iv) She showed a clear decrease in mental activity as a result of her second son's examination failure.
(v) Her second son announced his decision to go his own way, try to retake the examination, and leave home. During this period, although her mood gradually improved, her mental activity fluctuated sharply because of the sense of loss that occasionally struck her but gradually recovered after a while. Thereafter, there were no major events, and mental activity stabilized.
(vi) When the time came for her second son to take the entrance examinations again, and perhaps because she was worried about the results, her mental activity began to decrease again. Compared to a year earlier, her son no longer lived with her; she did not become too nervous or irritable and did not show dramatic fluctuations in her psychokinetic values.
(vii) With the good news that her second son had finished taking the examination and had passed it, her mental activity recovered.
(viii) Her pleasure was just for a short period as her third son, who had passed his matriculation examinations a year ago, clashed with the school and stopped attending, which made her mental activity dramatically decreasing at first and then continuing to fluctuate.
(ix) Her third son finally decided to quit school, announced his intention to lead an independent life, and left home. Immediately after this, her mental activity

showed a decrease but stabilized only after a week. She finally began embracing the days of peace.

As described above, the woman's data showed that the results of the voice-based MIMOSYS analysis were an accurate response to the events that occurred around her. She reported checking her state each time she used the MIMOSYS app and tried to change her thoughts and feelings accordingly. If her stress resilience skills were low, her mental activity would have remained dramatically low or even caused depression. This case study suggests that objective recognition of one's state of self using MIMOSYS is effective.

6.3 Case Study of Monitoring the Mental State of Elderly People

Rapidly aging societies are recognized as an important challenge in many countries. As retirement is delayed with increasing life expectancy, sustaining life motivation is important for extending healthy life expectancy. Therefore, the hypothesis that light work tasks improve Quality of Life (QoL) by maintaining and promoting life motivation in older adults was examined using the results of the MIMOSYS analysis (Nakamura et al. 2019).

Fifteen participants (five males and ten females) were recruited from the residents of the nursing home to participate in the study and provided informed consent. Participants in the experimental group performed light work on a sand cultivation farm, whereas those in the control group did not perform any light work. Audio recordings were made immediately before and after the light work in the experimental group. In the control group, audio recordings were performed twice at intervals corresponding to the time taken for the light work.

Vitality was analyzed from the audio recordings using the MIMOSYS algorithm as the soundness index at the time of recording, and the mean change in the soundness index before and after light work tasks or equivalent intervals for each group was compared.

As shown in Fig. 6.2, the mean change in the index of soundness before and after light work in the experimental group was greater than that in the control group, but this difference was not statistically significant, partly because the number of participants was limited, but a trend supporting the hypothesis could be observed.

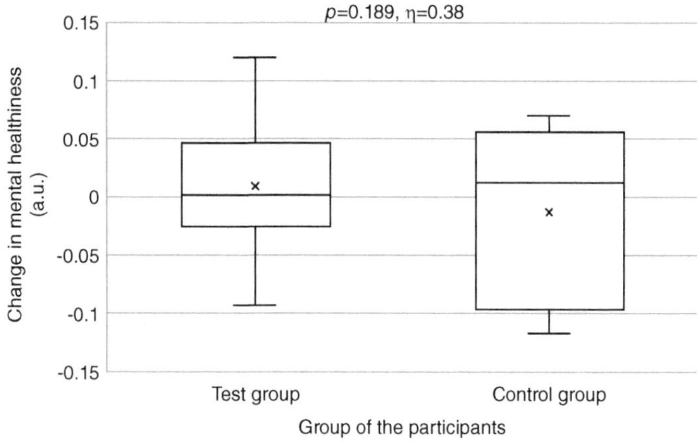

Fig. 6.2 Change between pre- and post-light work tasks

6.4 Case Study of Mental State Monitoring of Employees of a Company

Recently, overwork deaths and suicides among workers have become an undeniable issue, industrial health and medicine related to mental health have become important, and stress checks by employers have become obligatory with the revision of the Occupational Health and Safety Law. The usefulness of MIMOSYS in industrial settings for employees of cooperating companies was verified using technology to estimate mental health states by voice (Higuchi et al. 2018).

The subjects were 80 people (49 men and 31 women) who agreed to participate in the study and were asked to record their speech by reading standardized sentences at least once a day for 3 months from April to June 2017. Using this method, the mental health status at that time was analyzed as vitality, and the medium- and long-term mental health status as a mental activity. The company's own measurement data (weight, number of steps, blood pressure, and working hours of some employees) were matched to these data, and the frequency of measurement of each test, differences in results by department, and correlation trends between the data across time intervals were analyzed.

As a result, the measurement frequency of this method (at least one utterance per day) was approximately 50% at the beginning but decreased to 20% after approximately 1 month. The implementation rate of the company's own data on weight, blood pressure, and working hours, each of which required measurement using equipment installed in the office, remained approximately 20% each day since the beginning. The number of steps taken was consistently maintained at approximately 90%, probably because of the automatic measurement and transmission of results using portable devices.

Regarding the results of the analysis, there were no gender or age differences in the frequency of data measurement between our method and the company's data.

The frequency of measurements was higher for those who had been working for a shorter period. It was suggested that there may be a negative correlation between the length of working hours, vitality, and mental activity. There was a positive correlation between the number of steps taken and the mental activity. There was a slight positive correlation between the mean blood pressure, vitality, and mental activity.

These results suggest the need for a system for continuous measurement without a tiresome, as the frequency of measurement decreases and measurements that require some kind of action are likely to be carried out less frequently. In addition, it was reported that exercise reduces stress, and the positive correlation between stress, the number of steps, and mental activity in this study seems to be consistent. Although this case study suggests that the measurement of mental health status from voice is useful to some extent, it is also necessary to establish a system for continuous measurement.

6.5 Case Study of Mental State Monitoring of Newcomers

Omiya and Nagakawa reported a case study in which MIMOSYS was used to measure daily stress from the voice of new employees who were stressed by environmental changes (Omiya et al. 2017; Nagakawa and Tokuno 2018). The results were compared to those of the measurement of mental health status from voice using episodic information about the resignation offers of new employees with a high turnover rate.

In this study, and after asking for the consent of the subjects themselves, daily (weekdays only) voice stress measurements were conducted on approximately 1050 Japan Ground Self-Defense Forces members who participated in the study for approximately 3 months after the recruits' enlistment. Voice stress measurements were carried out using an Android OS smartphone with the MIMOSYS application installed. Moreover, the voice of 13 fixed phrases displayed on the screen was recorded, from which the short-term mental health status was measured as "vitality" and the long-term mental health status as "mental activity."

Figures 6.3, 6.4, 6.5, and 6.6 show four typical cases, mainly retirees who have experienced particularly strong stress.

For each case, a discussion of the relationship between the resignation offers an episodic information, and the results of the voice stress measurements are described below.

Case A: The participant's mental activity declined since the beginning of his enlistment, leading to his retirement. In a pre-retirement interview with an occupational physician, he suggested suiciding and was in a dangerous situation.

Case B: The participant's mental activity was low and stable from the beginning of his enlistment. Interviews with his supervisor indicated that he was unmotivated since the beginning of his enlistment, and his resignation was not considered a mental problem.

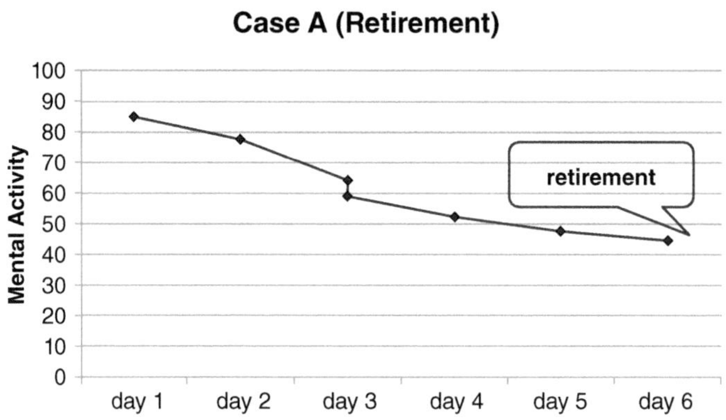

Fig. 6.3 Examples of changes in mental activity for newcomers (Case A)

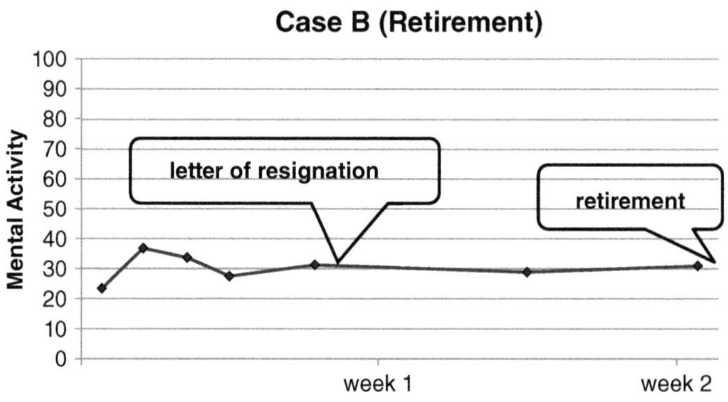

Fig. 6.4 Examples of changes in mental activity for newcomers (Case B)

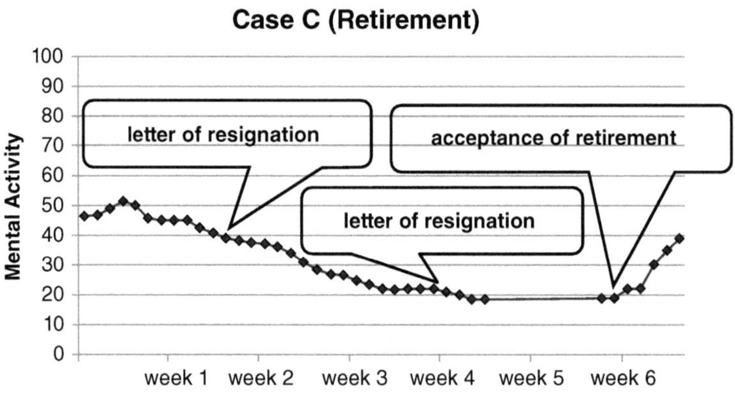

Fig. 6.5 Examples of changes in mental activity for newcomers (Case C)

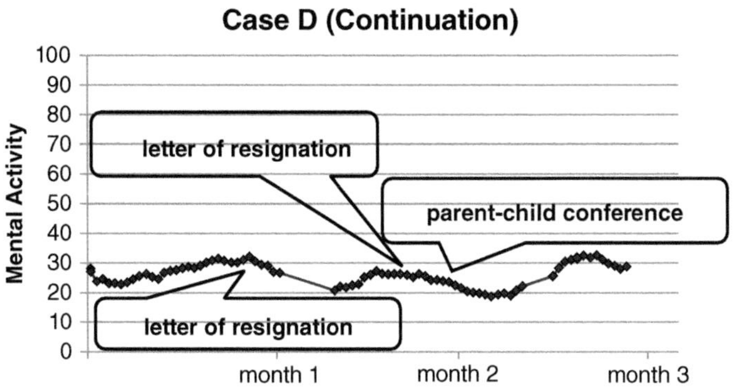

Fig. 6.6 Examples of changes in mental activity for newcomers (Case D)

Case C: The participant did not fit in with the organization and asked for resignation, but his supervisor persuaded him several times, and he accepted the persuasion, but his mental activity decreased. After resignation, the activity level recovered rapidly. It is thought that the person's true desire to quit was expressed in the mental activity, although superficially he agreed to persuasion.

Case D: The participant repeatedly asked to resign but was persuaded by his supervisor. Each time he was persuaded to stay, his mental activity decreased. The participant's true feelings were probably reflected in the mental activity, but after a certain period of time, the mental activity recovered, and with appropriate support and intervention, the patient had a positive attitude and did not resign.

In the Japan Ground Self-Defense Force, stress due to environmental changes accompanying enlistment was measured from voice using MIMOSYS, and trends in the measurement results were analyzed, mainly among retired personnel. As a result, interesting cases were found in which the person's mental health problems and their intention to retire were reflected in activity values. By detecting signs of mental disorders by voice stress measurements and taking early countermeasures, mental disorders can be prevented, which may lead to a reduction in the turnover rate.

6.6 Case Study of Kumamoto Earthquake Impact in a Large-Scale Social Implementation Research

During the data collection period of the large-scale social implementation study using MIMOSYS, a strong earthquake occurred with an epicenter in Kumamoto Prefecture, Japan, with an intensity of seven on the Japanese seismic scale. Figure 6.7 shows the changes in vitality 2 weeks before and after the earthquake in each region, and the values measured were averaged. After the earthquake, vitality decreased markedly in Shikoku, Kyushu, and Kumamoto.

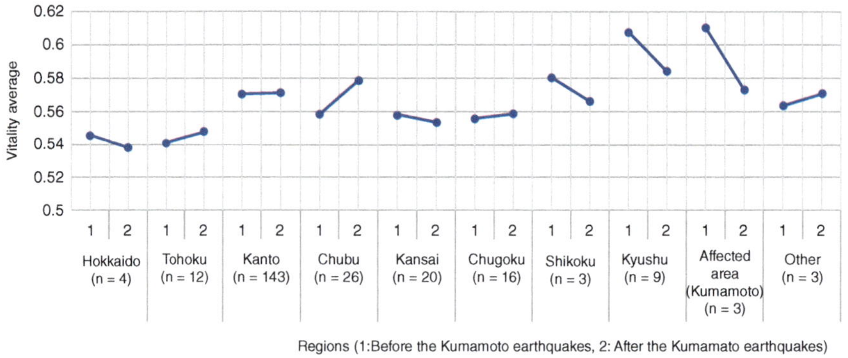

Fig. 6.7 Changes in vitality before and after the Kumamoto earthquakes. (Modified from Higuchi et al. 2020)

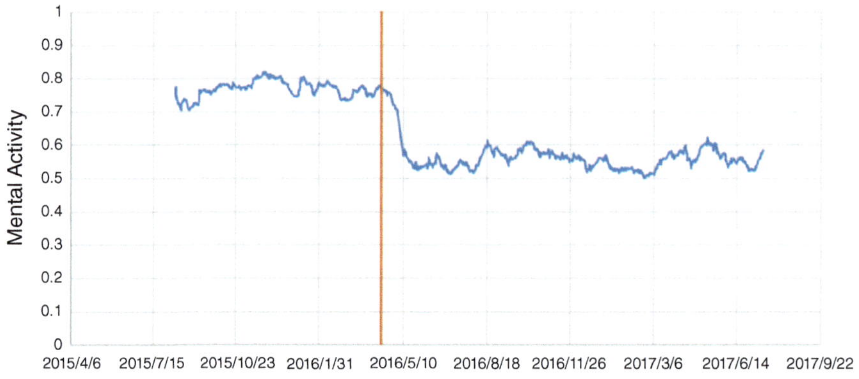

Fig. 6.8 Changes in mental activity of one of the victims of the Kumamoto earthquake. (Modified from Higuchi et al. 2020)

Figure 6.8 shows the change in mental activity over time for a single victim living in Kumamoto Prefecture. The vertical line in the graph indicates the foreshock date and time. There was an obvious decline in mental activity before and after the earthquake, and the latter did not return to their pre-earthquake levels before the end of the data collection period. One of the original purposes of MIMOSYS is to monitor and analyze changes in vitality and mental activity in relation to the user's life events. The results of the earthquake victims were the most obvious example of MIMOSYS detecting the stress caused by a life event. This suggests that MIMOSYS is a very effective monitoring system.

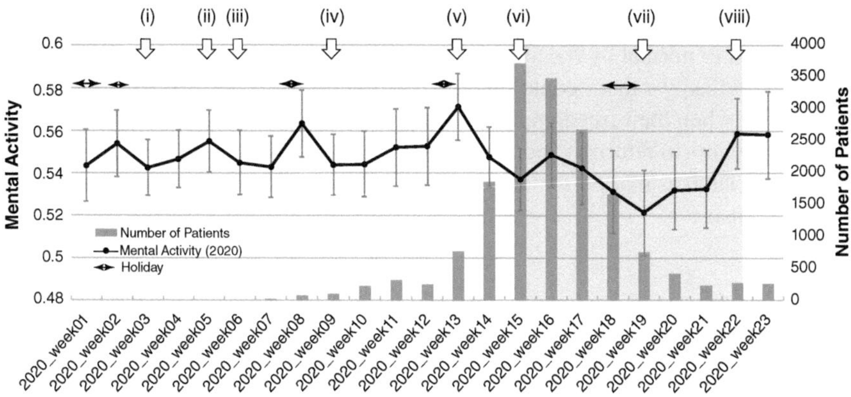

Fig. 6.9 Changes in mental activity due to COVID-19 pandemic. (Modified from Omiya and Tokuno 2020)(i) First case of infection reported in Japan. (ii) The charter plane brings 206 Japanese people back from Wuhan. (iii) The WHO declared a public health emergency, (iii) the WHO declared a public health emergency, and the quarantine of the Diamond Princess cruise ship began. (iv) Elementary, middle, and high schools were closed. (v) The governor of Tokyo mentioned a lockdown. (vi) State of emergency declared (voluntary isolation at home). (vii) The state of emergency extended. (viii) State of emergency is lifted

6.7 Case Study of COVID-19 Impact in a Large-Scale Social Implementation Research

Tokuno and Omiya reported the social impact of restricting going out following the COVID-19 epidemic (Tokuno 2020a, b; Omiya and Tokuno 2020).

The study covered the period from January 1 to June 6, 2020, and included 5246 MIMOSYS users, of which 126 were Japanese who continuously used the application's automatic call analysis function on their Android OS-based smartphones. Mental activity was calculated from the 2-week average of the results of the analysis of the vitality for one call and its variance. In this study, an analysis of three or more calls was made. The analysis results of 8669 calls by 90 users were used in the present study. The overall weekly mean and standard error were calculated from the weekly mean of each individual.

Figure 6.9 shows the psychological impact of COVID-19 "voluntary isolation at home" order in Japan. As shown in the figure, there was little decrease in mental activity during each of the pandemic-related episodes; rather, an increase was observed after the holiday, whereas a large decrease was observed by refraining from going out. Specifically, no changes were observed despite (1) reports of the first cases of infection in Japan, (2) the declaration of a state of emergency by the World Health Organization, (3) the start of quarantine on the Diamond Princess, and (4) requests to close primary, middle, and high schools. However, the decline in mental activity continued after the Governor of Tokyo referred to the lockdown, and the declaration of a state of emergency ("stay at home" order) further accelerated the decline in mental activity. However, as the termination date was indicated at the time of the extension of the emergency declaration, mental activity began to improve and returned to normal by the time the emergency declaration was lifted.

This trend shows that people react strongly to events that directly affect them, particularly when their freedom is restricted. The graph also shows a recovery trend when life begins to return to "normal," even if some freedom is absent. Analyses of the masses, such as that presented here, may be useful for policymaking in government and business.

6.8 Summary

We utilized MIMOSYS in various situations and found that it is effective for "objective recognition of one's own state," for "intervention and support by others" when objective recognition of one's own state does not lead to changes in one's own behavior, and for "group analysis and large-scale social implementation research." Case studies of group analysis and large-scale social implementation studies suggest that MIMOSYS is also effective for "monitoring a group of people" through events and light work. Furthermore, services using MIMOSYS (Yamashita 2018) are being developed as businesses, and expectations for MIMOSYS are increasing.

These results indicate that MIMOSYS is useful for monitoring people's mental health, although subjective methods such as questionnaires and interviews are generally used to serve the same purpose in the mental health field, not to mention that the introduction of speech indicators is expected.

References

Higuchi M, Miura Y, Shinohara S, Nakamura M, Omiya Y, Hagiwara N, Takano T, Mitsuyoshi S, Tokuno S (2018) Validation of voice-based mental health measurement for mental health care in industrial sites [Japanese]. In: The 91st annual meeting of the Japan Society for Occupational Health (Kumamoto), vol 5, pp 16–19

Higuchi M, Nakamura M, Shinohara S, Omiya Y, Takano T, Mitsuyoshi S, Tokuno S (2020) Effectiveness of a voice-based mental health evaluation system for JMIR. Form Res 4(7):e16455

Nagakawa M, Tokuno S (2018) Preventing turnover in new member education in the Japan ground self-defence force: the potential of mental health screening using speech analysis [Japanese]. In: The 57th annual conference of the Japanese Society for Medical and Biological Engineering (Sapporo), vol 6, pp 19–21

Nakamura M, Ikeuchi M, Oroguchi T, Yamanaka K, Amagi H, Shinohara S, Omiya Y, Higuchi M, Takano T, Mitsuyoshi S, Tokuno S (2019) Evaluation of the effect of light labour on retired people using voice analysis. In: 26th International "Stress and Behavior" neuroscience and biopsychiatry conference (ISBS 2019) (St. Petersburg), vol 5, pp 16–19

Omiya Y, Tokuno S (2020) How much of an impact did COVID-19 self-isolation measures have on mental health? Asian J Psychiatr 54:102445

Omiya Y, Hagiwara N, Nakamura M, Shinohara S, Higuchi M, Mitsuyoshi S, Toda H, Nagakawa M, Tokuno S (2017) An attempt to measure stress by voice for newly recruits in the Japan

Ground Self-Defence Force. In: The 90th annual meeting of the Japan Society for Occupational Health (Tokyo), vol 5, p 12
Tokuno S (2020a) Life events and voice biomarkers: voice analysis technology. Open Access Govern 2020(7):266–267
Tokuno S (2020b) Technology focus: social impact analysis using voice biomarkers. Open Access Govern 2020(10):184–185
Yamashita K (2018) Hitachi systems' approach to social implementation of MIMOSYS about Voice Kokoro Analysis Service. In: The 57th annual conference of the society for medical and biological engineering (Sapporo), vol 6, pp 19–21

Chapter 7
Depression: Jitter, Shimmer, Harmonic to Noise Ratio, and Pitch Rate

Shuji Shinohara

7.1 Introduction

Traditionally, jitter, shimmer, and harmonic noise ratio (HNR) have been used as indicators of periodic disturbances in voice. Whereas shimmer measures fluctuations in voice loudness, jitter measures fluctuations in voice pitch, which are affected by vocal fold tension and stiffness. HNR is an indicator of the stability of the harmonic structure and indicates the degree of voice disturbance, especially hoarseness. Figure 7.1 shows a schematic of the jitter and the shimmer. Jitter is a measure of how much each period T_i varies, and shimmer is a measure of how much each amplitude A_i varies. If perfectly periodic, both the jitter and shimmer would be zero.

Pitch is an indicator of voice tone. This index is calculated based on the assumption that voice is periodic. Jitter, shimmer, and HNR are indicators of periodicity disturbance, but they cannot be measured for parts of the data where the pitch is not detectable, that is, where there is no periodicity at all. Focusing on the ease of pitch detection, we propose using the pitch detection rate as an indicator of dysphonia. The pitch detection rate is defined as the percentage of frames in which pitch can be detected from all the frames to be analyzed.

While jitter and shimmer are indicators of small periodic disturbances within the range where the pitch can be detected, the pitch detection rate is an indicator of large periodic disturbances where the pitch cannot be detected. When the volume or pitch varies continuously, the jitter and shimmer are affected. However, fluctuations in volume or pitch do not affect the pitch detection rate as long as the fluctuations are small enough to detect the pitch. In other words, compared with jitter and

S. Shinohara (✉)
Division of Information Systems and Design, School of Science and Engineering, Tokyo Denki University, Hiki-gun, Saitama, Japan
e-mail: s.shinohara@mail.dendai.ac.jp

S. Tokuno, H. Nakamura (eds.), *Voice Biomarkers*,
https://doi.org/10.1007/978-981-96-3109-4_7

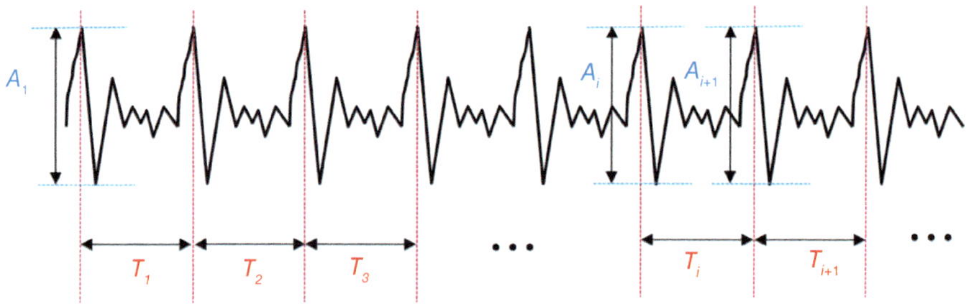

Fig. 7.1 Overview of jitter and shimmer. The figure represents a nearly periodic speech waveform, where T_i and A_i are the period and amplitude, respectively

shimmer, the pitch detection rate is a rough indicator and can be considered robust to fluctuations.

The purpose of this study was to discriminate between healthy subjects and patients using reading voices that are more similar to free speech than long vowels. Because free speech is more uncertain than long vowels, a rough measure, pitch detection rate, may be more appropriate for free speech. This study compares the effectiveness of pitch detection rate, jitter, shimmer, and harmonic noise ratio (HNR) as indicators of dysphonia using the long vowel "Ah" and English, German, and Japanese reading voices.

7.2 Voice Data

For English speech evaluation, we used the Disordered Voice Database and Program, Model 4337, from KayPENTAX, a division of Pentax Medical Inc. This database consists of approximately 700 long vowels "Ah" and English readings of the Rainbow Passage from healthy subjects and patients.

Long vowel data were collected from 53 healthy subjects and 658 patients, for a total of 711 subjects. However, jitter, shimmer, and HNR were not detected in 13 of the 658 patients' speech for long vowels. Therefore, 698 long vowels were used for the evaluation. Meanwhile, the reading voice data were collected from 53 healthy subjects and 662 patients for a total of 715 subjects.

The long vowel "Ah" is language independent. It is expected that there will be language differences in the words and pronunciations used in the reading of standardized sentences. In this study, we used English, Japanese, and German speech readings to evaluate the language dependence of each index.

For Germany, we used the "Saarbruecken Voice Database" (http://stimmdb.coli.uni-saarland.de/) from the Institute of Phonetics of Saarland University. This voice database contains data from more than 2000 individuals. In this study, the speech utterances "Guten morgen, wie geht es ihnen?" ("Good morning, how are you?")

for normal subjects and dysphonia patients were used for evaluation. These consisted of the speech of 632 normal subjects and 101 patients with dysphonia.

As for the Japanese, "Assessment of Motor Speech for Dysarthria" (Nishio 2009) was used. This speech database contains the speech of 6 normal subjects and 35 patients with dysarthria caused by various diseases. The speech was a reading of Aesop's fable "The North Wind and the Sun."

7.3 Evaluation Methods

Using the speech data described above, we calculated the pitch detection rate, jitter, shimmer, and HNR and compared the results between normal subjects and patients. To evaluate the discrimination performance between normal subjects and patients for each measure, we used the area under the curve (AUC) in the receiver operating characteristic (ROC) plot, along with the sensitivity and specificity. The t-test was used to test the differences between the means of each indicator. The significance level was set at 5%.

7.4 Voice Index

We used the speech analysis software Praat version 5.4.10 (http://www.fon.hum.uva.nl/praat/) to calculate jitter, shimmer, and HNR. In this study, we used ppq5 as the jitter, apq5 as the shimmer, and harmonicity as the HNR. In addition to these evaluation metrics, we introduced our pitch detection rate as a measure of speech impairment.

7.5 Pitch Detection Rate

Generally, there are silent intervals between utterances in recited speech. Pitch cannot be detected at these intervals. Therefore, the pitch detection rate was affected by the length of the silence intervals. For this reason, we used the Sensibility Technology software, version 3.0 (AGI Inc., Tokyo, Japan) (Mitsuyoshi et al. 2006, 2007; Mitsuyoshi 2002) to remove the silent intervals before calculating the pitch detection rate.

After the silent intervals were removed, the audio data were divided into frames of length L. However, the start of each frame was shifted from the previous frame by L/4. In other words, 3/4 of each frame overlaps with the previous frame. In this study, $L = 46.44$ ms. This corresponds to 512 data points at a sampling rate of 11,025 Hz.

Pitch was calculated using the following method (Mitsuyoshi 2006; Mitsuyoshi et al. 2002): First, a Fourier transform was applied to the signal waveform (Fig. 7.2a). The autocorrelation was calculated using the Fourier spectrum (Fig. 7.2b) to detect the peaks. Each peak was assigned a sequential number, and the position of each peak (F1, F1, F3, …), that is, the frequency shift ΔFrequency, was identified (Fig. 7.2c). The peak number was then plotted on the horizontal axis and Δ frequency on the vertical axis, and the regression line $Y = \alpha X + \beta$ was calculated (Fig. 7.2d). If the coefficient of determination R in the single regression analysis is

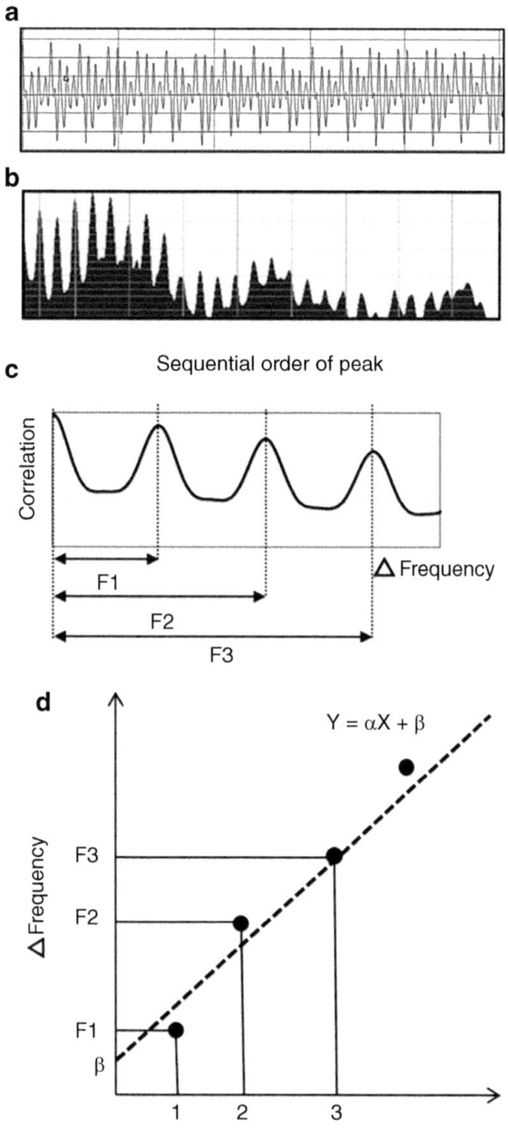

Fig. 7.2 Overview of the pitch extraction algorithm. (Modified from Shinohara et al. 2017)

greater than the threshold θ1 and the y-intercept β is less than the threshold θ2, then a pitch is detected from that frame, as expressed in Eq. (7.1).

$$\text{pitch} = \begin{cases} 1(\text{Detected}) & \text{if } R > \theta_1 \text{ and} |\beta| < \theta_2 \\ 0(\text{not Detected}) \text{otherwise} \end{cases} \tag{7.1}$$

If pitch is detected, the slope α of the regression line is the pitch.

The pitch detection rate is defined as the percentage of frames in the speech segment in which the pitch is detected. After the pitch detection rate was calculated for each utterance segment, the average pitch detection rate for all utterances in the voice file was calculated and used as the pitch detection rate for the voice in the file.

7.6 Results

7.6.1 Pitch Detection Rate, Jitter, Shimmer, and Harmonic Noise Ratio (HNR) Discrimination Performance for Long Vowels

For the pitch detection rate, the mean values for healthy subjects and patients were 0.99 (n = 53, standard deviation (SD) = 0.0049) and 0.84 (n = 645, SD = 0.26), respectively. The t-test results showed a significant difference between the two ($t(695) = 14.55$, $p = 7.55 \bullet 10^{-42}$).

For jitter, the mean values for healthy participants and patients were 0.0016 (n = 53, SD = 0.00066) and 0.0061 (n = 645, SD = 0.0078), respectively. The t-test results showed a significant difference between the two ($t(695) = -14.05$, $p = 1.23 \bullet 10^{-39}$).

For shimmer, the mean values for the healthy subjects and patients were 0.012 (n = 53, SD = 0.0062) and 0.039 (n = 645, SD = 0.0293), respectively. The t-test results showed a significant difference between the two ($t(329) = -19.01$, $p = 7.04 \bullet 10^{-55}$).

For HNR, the mean values for healthy subjects and patients were 23.94 (n = 53, SD = 2.86) and 15.18 (n = 645, SD = 6.19), respectively. The t-test results showed a significant difference between the two ($t(97) = 18.77$, $p = 4.76 \bullet 10^{-34}$). The results are summarized in Table 7.1.

Table 7.1 Mean values for healthy individuals and patients in the data of the long vowel sound "Ah"

Index	Healthy individuals (n = 53)	Patients (n = 645)	P-value
Pitch detection rate	0.99 ± 0.0049	0.84 ± 0.26	$7.55 \bullet 10^{-42}$
Jitter (ppq5)	0.0016 ± 0.00066	0.0061 ± 0.0078	$1.23 \bullet 10^{-39}$
Shimmer (apq5)	0.012 ± 0.0062	0.039 ± 0.0293	$7.04 \bullet 10^{-55}$
HNR (harmonicity)	23.94 ± 2.86	15.18 ± 6.19	$4.76 \bullet 10^{-34}$

Figure 7.3 shows the ROC curves when these indices were used to discriminate between the healthy subjects and patients. The abscissa represents 1-specificity (false-positive rate), and the ordinate represents sensitivity (true-positive rate). Table 7.2 presents the AUC, sensitivity, and specificity of each index. The AUC for all indices was approximately 0.9 or higher, indicating a very high discrimination performance. In particular, the pitch detection rate showed the highest discrimination performance with an AUC of 0.981.

7.6.2 Discrimination Performance of Pitch Detection Rate, Jitter, Shimmer, and HNR for the English Reading of "Rainbow Passage"

For the pitch detection rate, the mean values for the healthy subjects and patients were 0.903 ($n = 53$, SD = 0.047) and 0.643 ($n = 662$, SD = 0.25), respectively. The t-test results showed a significant difference between them ($t(394) = 22.285$, $p = 8.98 \bullet 10^{-39}$).

For jitter, the mean values for the healthy subjects and patients were 0.0084 ($n = 53$, SD = 0.0016) and 0.014 ($n = 662$, SD = 0.0076), respectively. The t-test results showed a significant difference between the two groups ($t(321) = -15.09$, $p = 2.84 \bullet 10^{-39}$).

For shimmer, the mean values for the healthy subjects and patients were 0.042 ($n = 53$, SD = 0.010) and 0.057 ($n = 662$, SD = 0.026), respectively. The t-test results showed a significant difference between the two groups ($t(117) = -8.58$, $p = 4.55 \bullet 10^{-14}$).

For HNR, the mean values for healthy subjects and patients were 13.12 ($n = 53$, SD = 2.18) and 11.41 ($n = 662$, SD = 3.48), respectively. The t-test results showed

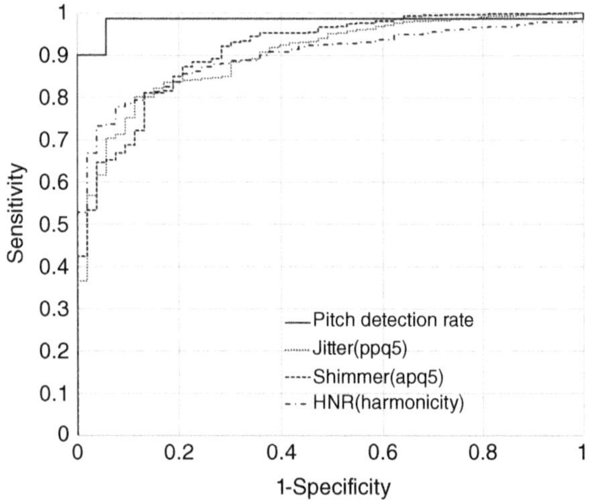

Fig. 7.3 Receiver operating characteristic (ROC) curves for the long vowel "Ah" using pitch detection rate, jitter, shimmer, and harmonic noise ratio (HNR) to discriminate between healthy subjects and patients. (Modified from Shinohara et al. 2017)

Table 7.2 Discrimination performance of each index for the long vowel "Ah" between healthy subjects and patients

Index	Area under the curve (AUC)	Sensitivity	Specificity
Pitch detection rate	0.981	0.986	0.943
Jitter (ppq5)	0.900	0.802	0.887
Shimmer (apq5)	0.911	0.811	0.868
HNR (harmonicity)	0.897	0.778	0.925

Table 7.3 Mean values for healthy individuals and patients in the data of the read speech of "Rainbow Passage"

Index	Healthy individuals ($n = 53$)	Patients ($n = 662$)	P-value
Pitch detection rate	0.903 ± 0.047	0.643 ± 0.25	$8.98 \cdot 10^{-39}$
Jitter (ppq5)	0.0084 ± 0.0016	0.014 ± 0.0076	$2.84 \cdot 10^{-39}$
Shimmer (apq5)	0.042 ± 0.010	0.057 ± 0.026	$4.55 \cdot 10^{-14}$
HNR (harmonicity)	13.12 ± 2.18	11.41 ± 3.48	$1.91 \cdot 10^{-6}$

a significant difference between the two (($t(75) = 5.166, p = 1.91 \cdot 10^{-6}$). The results are summarized in Table 7.3.

Figure 7.4 shows the ROC curves for the case in which each index was used to discriminate between normal subjects and patients. The horizontal axis represents 1-specificity (false-positive rate), and the vertical axis represents sensitivity (true-positive rate). Table 7.4 presents the AUC, sensitivity, and specificity of each indicator.

Compared to Table 7.2, it can be observed that the discrimination performance was reduced for all indicators compared to that in the case of long vowels. The degree of decline was particularly significant for shimmer and HNR.

7.6.3 Discrimination Performance of Pitch Detection Rate, Jitter, Shimmer, and HNR for the German Recitation of "Guten morgen, wie geht es ihnen?"

For the pitch detection rate, the mean values for the healthy subjects and patients were 0.826 (n = 632, SD = 0.094) and 0.701 (n = 101, SD = 0.180), respectively. The t-test results showed a significant difference between the two groups ($t(109) = 6.78, p = 6.55 \cdot 10^{-10}$).

For jitter, the mean values for the healthy subjects and patients were 0.0101 (n = 632, SD = 0.0028) and 0.0122 (n = 101, SD = 0.0056), respectively. The t-test results showed a significant difference between the two ($t(632) = -3.66$, $p = 3.90 \cdot 10^{-4}$).

For shimmer, the mean values for healthy subjects and patients were 0.036 (n = 632, SD = 0.012) and 0.045 (n = 101, SD = 0.019), respectively. The t-test

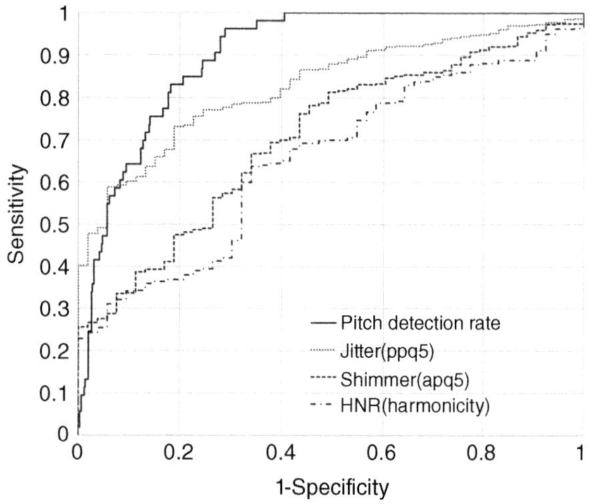

Fig. 7.4 ROC curves for the discrimination between normal subjects and patients using pitch detection rate, jitter, shimmer, and HNR for the English reading of "Rainbow Passage." (Modified from Shinohara et al. 2017)

Table 7.4 Discrimination performance of each index between normal subjects and patients for the English reading of "Rainbow Passage"

Index	AUC	Sensitivity	Specificity
Pitch detection rate	0.902	0.962	0.713
Jitter (ppq5)	0.827	0.588	0.943
Shimmer (apq5)	0.706	0.761	0.566
HNR (harmonicity)	0.655	0.636	0.660

results showed a significant difference between the two ($t(112) = -4.25$, $p = 4.48 \cdot 10^{-5}$).

For HNR, the mean values for healthy subjects and patients were 14.89 ($n = 632$, SD = 2.29) and 14.47 ($n = 101$, SD = 3.27), respectively. The t-test results showed no significant difference between the two ($t(116) = 1.230$, $p = 0.22$). Table 7.5 summarizes the results.

Figure 7.5 shows the ROC curves for discrimination between healthy subjects and patients using each index. The abscissa represents 1-specificity (false-positive rate), and the ordinate represents sensitivity (true-positive rate). Table 7.6 presents the AUC, sensitivity, and specificity of each indicator.

The pitch detection rate performance was the best for AUC. However, the overall discrimination performance was lower than that in English.

Table 7.5 Mean values for healthy individuals and patients in the data of the read speech of "Guten morgen, wie geht es ihnen?"

Index	Healthy individuals (n = 632)	Patients (n = 101)	P-value
Pitch rate	0.826 ± 0.094	0.701 ± 0.180	$6.55 \bullet 10^{-10}$
Jitter (ppq5)	0.0101 ± 0.0028	0.0122 ± 0.0056	0.00039
Shimmer (apq5)	0.036 ± 0.012	0.045 ± 0.019	$4.48 \bullet 10^{-5}$
HNR (harmonicity)	14.89 ± 2.29	14.47 ± 3.27	0.22

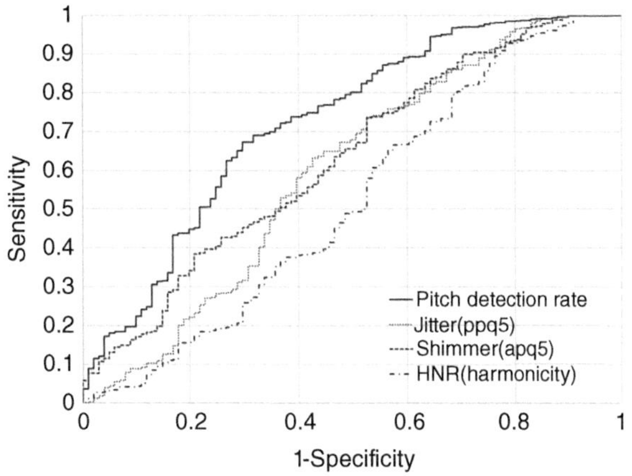

Fig. 7.5 ROC curves for the German reading "Guten morgen, wie geht es ihnen?" using pitch detection rate, jitter, shimmer, and HNR to discriminate between normal subjects and patients. (Modified from Shinohara et al. 2017)

7.6.4 Discrimination Performance of Pitch Detection Rate, Jitter, Shimmer, and HNR for the Japanese Recitation of "Kitakaze to Taiyo (The North Wind and the Sun)"

For speech duration, the mean values for normal subjects and patients were 26144.17 ms (n = 6, SD = 2995.73) and 18676.11 ms (n = 35, SD = 5145.64), respectively.

For the pitch detection rate, the mean values for healthy subjects and patients were 0.831 (n = 6, SD = 0.051) and 0.668 (n = 35, SD = 0.232), respectively. The t-test results showed a significant difference between the two groups ($t(36) = 3.67$, $p = 7.80 \bullet 10^{-4}$).

For jitter, the mean values for the healthy subjects and patients were 0.011 (n = 6, SD = 0.0026) and 0.013 (n = 35, SD = 0.0084), respectively. The t-test results showed no significant difference between the two groups ($t(26) = -1.61$, $p = 1.20 \bullet 10^{-1}$).

For shimmer, the mean values for healthy subjects and patients were 0.040 (n = 6, SD = 0.014) and 0.062 (n = 35, SD = 0.035), respectively. The t-test results showed a significant difference between the two ($t(19) = -2.76$, $p = 1.30 \bullet 10^{-2}$).

For HNR, the means for healthy subjects and patients were 13.64 (n = 6, SD = 2.46) and 11.85 (n = 35, SD = 3.59), respectively. The t-test results showed no significant difference between the two groups ($t(39) = 1.17$, $p = 2.50 \bullet 10^{-1}$). Table 7.7 summarizes the results.

Table 7.6 Discrimination performance of each index between healthy subjects and patients for the German reading of "Guten morgen, wie geht es ihnen?"

Index	AUC	Sensitivity	Specificity
Pitch detection rate	0.725	0.672	0.703
Jitter (ppq5)	0.598	0.734	0.475
Shimmer (apq5)	0.628	0.736	0.475
HNR (harmonicity)	0.519	0.927	0.218

Table 7.7 Mean values for healthy individuals and patients in the data of the read speech of "Kitakaze to Taiyo"

Index	Healthy individuals ($n = 6$)	Patients ($n = 35$)	P-value
Pitch detection rate	0.831 ± 0.051	0.668 ± 0.232	$7.80 \cdot 10^{-4}$
Jitter (ppq5)	0.011 ± 0.0026	0.013 ± 0.0084	$1.20 \cdot 10^{-1}$
Shimmer (apq5)	0.040 ± 0.014	0.0625 ± 0.035	$1.30 \cdot 10^{-2}$
HNR (harmonicity)	13.64 ± 2.46	11.85 ± 3.59	$2.50 \cdot 10^{-1}$

Figure 7.6 shows the ROC curves for discrimination between healthy subjects and patients using each index. The abscissa shows 1-specificity (false-positive rate), and the ordinate shows sensitivity (true-positive rate). Table 7.8 presents the AUC, sensitivity, and specificity of each index.

The pitch detection rate performance was the best for AUC. However, as in the German case, the overall discrimination performance was lower than that in the English case.

7.7 Discussion

In this study, we propose a method to discriminate between normal subjects and patients with dysphonia using the pitch detection rate of speech segments.

We evaluated the discriminative performance of pitch detection rate using long vowels and speech readings in English, German, and Japanese and compared it to jitter, shimmer, and HNR. Similar studies have compared healthy subjects and patients using the same speech samples (Al-Nasheri et al. 2017), but these studies used long vowel speech. This study analyzed not only long vowels but also recited speech. As presented in Table 7.2, for long vowels, the pitch detection rate, jitter, shimmer, and HNR showed discrimination performance with AUCs of almost 0.9 or better. In particular, the pitch detection rate exhibited the best performance with an AUC of 0.98. However, as indicated in Table 7.4, the discrimination performance for all indices decreased for the English read speech. The decrease in AUC was particularly pronounced for shimmer and HNR, reaching approximately 0.7. Meanwhile, the AUC of the pitch detection rate was above 0.9 for the recited speech. Thus, in the case of English speech, the discrimination performance of the pitch

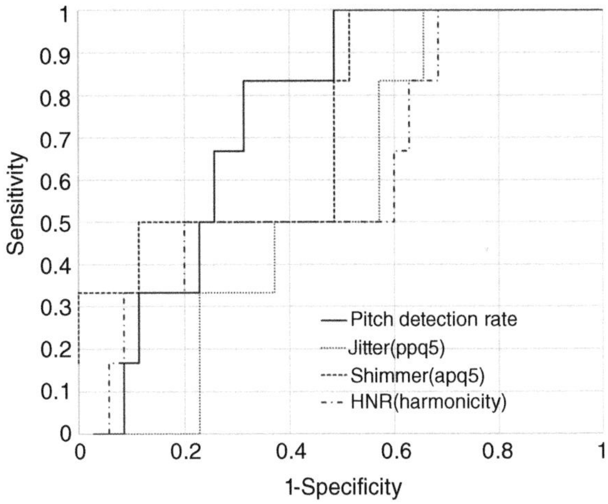

Fig. 7.6 ROC curves for the Japanese reading "Kitakaze to Taiyo" using pitch detection rate, jitter, shimmer, and HNR to discriminate between normal subjects and patients. (Modified from Shinohara et al. 2017)

Table 7.8 Discrimination performance of each index between normal subjects and patients for the Japanese reading of "Kitakaze to Taiyo"

Index	AUC	Sensitivity	Specificity
Pitch detection rate	0.752	0.833	0.686
Jitter (ppq5)	0.562	1.00	0.343
Shimmer (apq5)	0.733	1.00	0.486
HNR (harmonicity)	0.624	1.00	0.314

detection rate is the best compared with conventional indices for both long vowels and recited speech.

The best discriminative performance for pitch detection rate was also observed for German and Japanese read speech. However, for all measures, the AUC was lower than that in English. In the case of English speech reading, the pitch detection rates for normal subjects and patients were 0.903 and 0.643, respectively. In contrast, for German speech reading, the pitch detection rates for healthy subjects and patients were 0.826 and 0.701, respectively. For the Japanese reading, the pitch detection rates for the healthy subjects and patients were 0.831 and 0.668, respectively. In other words, pitch detection rates were lower for normal subjects and higher for patients in German and Japanese than in English. The difference in pitch detection rates in healthy subjects may be due to differences in speech content and language. The difference in the pitch detection rate for patients may be due to the severity of dysphonia in patients in the database.

In the case of German, speech is a greeting used in daily life that can be spoken naturally without reading. This may affect the pitch detection rate.

As described in Sect. 7.2, two threshold values, θ1 and θ2, were used to calculate the pitch detection rate, and the same values were used for each language in this evaluation. Although not shown here, when the optimal threshold values were set for each language, the AUC exceeded 0.8 for both German and Japanese read speech.

The pitch detection rate showed the highest discrimination performance for long and recited vowels. It should be noted, however, that our ultimate goal is to obtain high discrimination performance in free speech and that recited speech is different from free speech. In this study, the same phrases were used to compare pitch detection rates between healthy subjects and patients. However, in everyday speech, the content of the speech is diverse and differs each time. For example, the more consonants in an utterance, the lower the pitch detection rate. The effect of speech content on the pitch detection rate and the difference in discrimination performance between recited and free speech should be analyzed in the future.

For pitch extraction, we used the method proposed in the literature (Mitsuyoshi 2006; Mitsuyoshi et al. 2002). There are various methods for pitch extraction, and the pitch value itself may change if other methods are used. However, the pitch detection rate represents whether a pitch is detected and is independent of the pitch value. Therefore, as long as the same method is used for pitch extraction of the speech of healthy subjects and patients, it is expected that similar results will be obtained, regardless of the method used.

References

Al-Nasheri A, Muhammad G, Alsulaiman M, Ali Z, Mesallam TA, Farahat M, Malki KH, Bencherif MA (2017) An investigation of multidimensional voice program parameters in three different databases for voice pathology detection and classification. J Voice 31(1):113.e9–113.e18

Mitsuyoshi S (2002) Emotion recognizing method, sensibility creating method, device, and software. WO0223524

Mitsuyoshi S (2006) Research on the phonetic recognition of feelings and a system for emotional physiological brain signal analysis. PhD thesis, Tokushima University, Tokushima

Mitsuyoshi S, Ogata K, Monma F (2002) Speech analyzer detecting pitch frequency, speech analyzing method, and speech analyzing program. WO2006132159

Mitsuyoshi S, Ren F, Tanaka Y, Kuroiwa S (2006) Non-verbal voice emotion analysis system. Int J Innov Comput Inf Control 2(4):819–830

Mitsuyoshi S, Tanaka Y, Ren F, Shibasaki K, Kato M, Murata T, Minami T, Yagura H (2007) Emotion voice analysis system connected to the human brain. In: IEEE NLP-KE 2007, pp 479–484

Nishio M (2009) Assessment of motor speech for dysarthria. Interuna Publishers, Inc. ISBN 978-4-900637-38-2 (in Japanese)

Shinohara S, Omiya Y, Nakamura M, Hagiwara N, Higuchi M, Mitsuyoshi S, Tokuno S (2017) Multilingual evaluation of voice disability index using pitch rate. Adv Sci Technol Eng Syst 2(3):765–772

Chapter 8
Depression: Our Original Features

Shuji Shinohara

8.1 Introduction

In recent years, with the progress of neuroscience research, the link between depression and arousal has attracted attention. Many studies have been conducted using physiological indices such as EEG (e.g., late positive potential (LPP) amplitude), magnetoencephalography (e.g., neuromagnetic oscillatory activity), skin conductance, and other physiological indicators (Schmidt et al. 2017; Moratti et al. 2008; Benning and Ait 2017).

Benning and Ait Oumeziane (2017) suggested that low arousal and low positive emotion may be core affective components of potential depression through studies using physiological indicators, such as LPP amplitude and skin conductance. In addition, in the Diagnostic and Statistical Manual of Mental Disorders, Fourth Edition, Text Revision (DSM-IV-TR), major depression is characterized by episodes of decreased interest and pleasure, sadness, and emptiness (American Psychiatric Association 2000). In terms of speech, depressed patients have been reported to be dull, monotonous, and lifeless (Sobin and Sackeim 1997). Methods used to assess emotional arousal from speech have been studied. The relationships between arousal and vocal intensity and pitch have also been tested (Bone et al. 2014; Schmidt et al. 2016).

Based on these findings, we hypothesized that the voices of patients with depression would tend to have lower levels of arousal. Based on this hypothesis, we aimed to first calculate emotional arousal from voice and then use the voice arousal index to assess depression rather than directly detecting depression from voice features. First, we used emotional speech stored in the interactive emotional dyadic motion

S. Shinohara (✉)
Division of Information Systems and Design, School of Science and Engineering, Tokyo Denki University, Hiki-gun, Saitama, Japan
e-mail: s.shinohara@mail.dendai.ac.jp

S. Tokuno, H. Nakamura (eds.), *Voice Biomarkers*,
https://doi.org/10.1007/978-981-96-3109-4_8

capture (IEMOCAP) database (Busso et al. 2008) to construct two algorithms for calculating emotional arousal from speech. One study used the relationship between the Hurst exponent (HE) and the zero crossing rate (ZCR) of the speech waveform. The other used the acceleration of the change in the sound pressure. These algorithms were then used to extract emotional arousal from the speeches of patients with depression. Finally, the relationship between these measures and depression severity based on the Hamilton Rating Scale for Depression (HAM-D) was examined.

8.2 Measurement of Emotional Arousal by Voice

8.2.1 Emotional Speech Data

We used the IEMOCAP database (Busso et al. 2008) to create and validate an algorithm for calculating emotional arousal from the acoustic features of voices. The database contains dialogues for five male–female pairs. Each dialogue was manually segmented into speech units containing 10039 utterances. The arousal level of each utterance was rated by two annotators on a five-point scale, with the average value being the arousal level of each utterance. Cronbach's alpha coefficients (Cronbach 1951) were computed to test the reliability of the evaluations between raters. Coefficient was 0.607.

In addition, the emotion of each utterance was assessed using at least three annotators. The emotions addressed were "angry," "happy," "sad," "neutral," "frustrated," "excited," "fearful," "surprised," and "disgusted." Too many emotion categories resulted in low inter-rater agreement. However, too few of them will result in a less accurate representation of emotions. To balance this trade-off, IEMOCAP uses the basic emotions known as "anger," "sadness," "happiness," "disgust," "fear," and "surprise" (Ekman and Friesen 1971), plus "frustration," "excitement," and "neutral" as the nine emotion categories selected. However, during the evaluation, utterances that did not seem to fit into any of these categories were classified as "other." Where there was disagreement between the annotators regarding classification, a simple majority voting method was used to assign emotion categories. Annotators were allowed to tag more than one emotion category. If the majority vote did not result in a category, that category was labelled xxx. This procedure resulted in 7527 utterances out of 10,039 utterances assigned to the 9 emotion categories. To analyze the degree of agreement between raters, the Fleiss' kappa statistic (Fleiss 1981) was calculated, with a value of $\kappa = 0.27$.

Figure 8.1 shows the number of utterances classified into each emotional category. The numbers of the three categories "fearful," "surprised," and "disgusted" are extremely low compared to the other categories. The number (percentage) of utterances in these three categories was 40 (0.53%), 103 (1.42%), and 2 (0.03%), respectively.

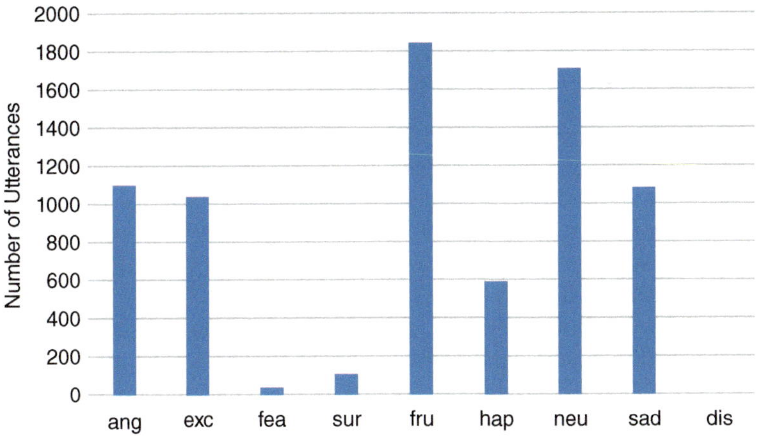

Fig. 8.1 The number of utterances for each emotion category. (Modified from Shinohara et al. 2021)
Note: The number of utterances classified in "disgusted" was 2. In addition, ang angry, exc excited, *fea* fearful, *sur* surprised, *fru* frustrated, *hap* happy, *neu* neutral, *sad* sad, and *dis* disgusted

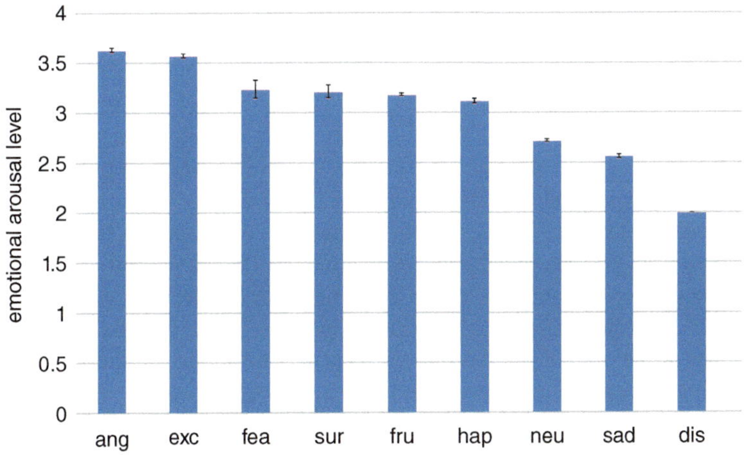

Fig. 8.2 The mean emotional arousal level for each emotion category
Note: Error bars represent standard error. In addition, *ang* angry, *exc* excited, *fea* fearful, *sur* surprised, *fru* frustrated, *hap* happy, *neu* neutral, *sad* sad, and *dis* disgusted. (Modified from Shinohara et al. 2021)

Figure 8.2 shows the mean emotional arousal values for utterances classified into each emotional category. However, the emotional categories on the horizontal axis are aligned in the order of the highest mean emotional arousal value. As can be seen from the figure, emotional arousal is higher in the categories "angry" and "excited" and lower in the categories "neutral," "sad," and "disgusted." This seems to be in line with our everyday perceptions. In addition, "fearful," "surprised," "frustrated," and "happy" did not show much difference in emotional arousal.

8.2.2 Emotional Arousal Index Using the Hurst Exponent and Zero Crossing Rate

In this section, we introduce an emotional arousal voice index using two features Hurst exponent (HE) and zero crossing rate (ZCR) (Shinohara et al. 2020).

We used low arousal data with arousal levels of 2 or lower (n = 1112, arousal mean ± standard deviation SD = 1.92 ± 0.19) and high arousal data with arousal levels of 4 or higher (n = 1692, arousal mean 4.19 ± SD = 0.28) from all 10,039 utterances in IEMOCAP to create this index.

HE is widely used in the field of stock price analysis to measure the long-term memory characteristics of a time series (Eom et al. 2008). First, the difference in $\Delta x(t,\tau) = x(t+\tau) - x(t)$ between signal $x(t)$ at time t and signal $x(t+\tau)$ after τ is determined. The standard deviation $\sigma(\tau)$ of the time-series data $\Delta x(t,\tau)$ is then obtained as follows:

$$\sigma(\tau) = \sqrt{\frac{\sum_{t=1}^{n-\tau}\left(\Delta x(t,\tau) - \overline{\Delta x(\tau)}\right)^2}{n-\tau-1}}$$

$$\Delta x(t,\tau) = x(t+\tau) - x(t)$$

$$\overline{\Delta x(\tau)} = \frac{\sum_{t=1}^{n}\Delta x(t,\tau)}{n} \tag{8.1}$$

It is known that a power relation ($\sigma(\tau) \propto \tau^{\alpha}$ or $\log(\sigma(\tau)) \propto \alpha \log(\tau)$) exists between $\sigma(\tau)$ and τ when τ is small and the exponent α is called HE. We set the range of τ in determining HE to be $\tau \leq 1.46$ ms. For example, if the sampling frequency of the speech data is 11,025 Hz, this range corresponds to 16 data points.

The specific calculation method is to first vary τ from τ = 1/11025 s to τ = 16/11025 s and calculate the $\sigma(\tau)$ for each τ. Then, we take the logarithm $(\log(\tau), \log(\sigma(\tau)))$ of $(\tau, \sigma(\tau))$ and use all 16 points to obtain a regression line. The slope of this regression line was defined as HE. However, if the coefficient of determination is less than 0.9 when the regression line is calculated, it is assumed that the power–law relationship does not hold, and the value of HE is invalid.

Theoretically, HE is HE = 0.0 for white noise and HE = 0.5 for brown noise; for smooth waveforms such as sin waves, HE is close to 1.0; when D is the fractal dimension of the signal waveform, HE is expressed as HE = 2 − D. In other words, HE can be regarded as an indicator of the smoothness of the waveform (inverse of the fractal dimension).

In contrast, ZCR is an index commonly used in studies on voice activity detection and voiced/unvoiced sound classification, which indicates the rate at which the signal changes from positive to negative or vice versa (Jalil et al. 2013; Bachu et al. 2010; Kazi et al. 2017). Specifically, the ZCR of a signal, which is a signal of length n, is calculated as

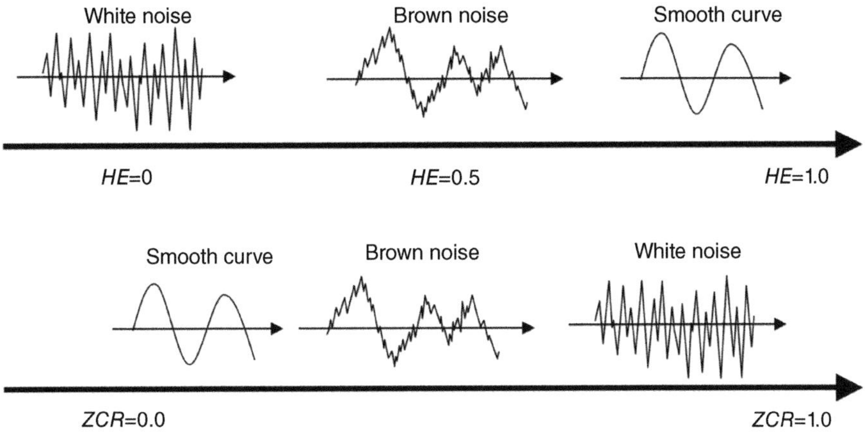

Fig. 8.3 The rough relationship between HE, ZCR, and waveform

$$
\begin{aligned}
ZCR &= \frac{\sum_{t=1}^{n-1} I(y(t)y(t+1))}{n-1} \\
y(t) &= x(t) - \overline{x} \\
\overline{x} &= \frac{\sum_{t=1}^{n} x(t)}{n} \\
I(y(t)y(t+1)) &= \begin{cases} 1 & if\ y(t)y(t+1) < 0 \\ 0 & else \end{cases}
\end{aligned}
\tag{8.2}
$$

where $\overline{x}$ is the average value of $x(t)$, and $y(t)$ is the value corrected for $x(t)$, so that the average is 0. ZCR, in contrast to HE, is smaller for smooth waveforms and larger for white noise. The rough relationship between HE, ZCR, and the waveform is shown in Fig. 8.3.

We focused on the relationship between HE and ZCR as a voice index of arousal. First, the utterance is divided into frames of length L. However, each frame is set to overlap its neighboring frame by L/4. In this study, L was set to 46.44 ms. At a sampling frequency of 11,025 Hz, this corresponded to 512 data points. The HE and ZCR were then calculated for each frame. Next, only the frames in the utterance for which the HE values were valid were selected. The average HE and ZCR values of these frames were taken as the HE and ZCR of the utterance.

Figure 8.4 shows a scatterplot of HE and ZCR calculated from utterances in the IEMOCAP database. Here, the speech data with arousal level below 2 are considered low-arousal data (n = 1112) and the data with arousal level above 4 are considered high-arousal data (n = 1692), and only these data are displayed. The figure shows that as HE increases, the ZCR tends to become smaller. Furthermore, it can be seen that the high-arousal data appear higher than the low-arousal data.

Here, we performed a logistic regression analysis to classify the low- and high-arousal data. In this analysis, the explanatory variables were HE and ZCR. However,

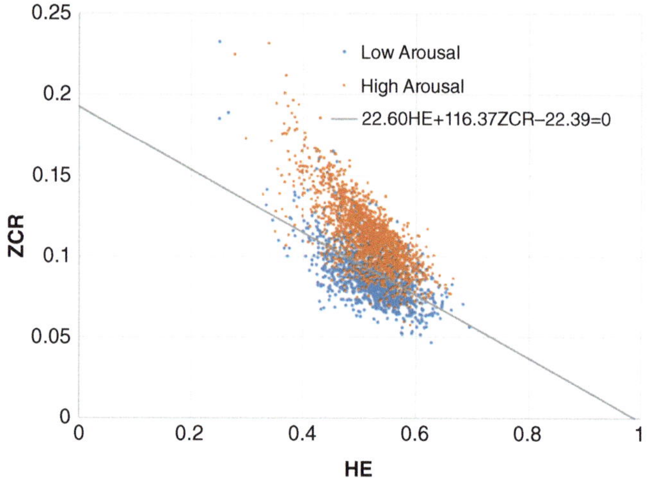

Fig. 8.4 Scatterplot of HE and ZCR calculated from utterances in the IEMOCAP database. (Modified from Shinohara et al. 2020)

we assigned a dummy variable of 0 to the low-arousal data and 1 to the high-arousal data. These two values were used as the objective variables. The discriminant score obtained from this logistic regression analysis is referred to as arousal-level voice index 1 (ALVI1) in this study.

$$\mathrm{ALVI1} = \frac{1}{1 + \exp\left[-\left(21.60\mathrm{HE} + 116.37\mathrm{ZCR} - 22.39\right)\right]} \tag{8.3}$$

ALVI1 takes values in the range (0.0, 1.0). A straight line 21.60HE + 116.37ZCR − 22.39 = 0, which lines up the group of points where ALVI1 = 0.5, is also shown in Fig. 8.4. The mean ALVI1 values for the low- and high-arousal groups were 0.33 ± 0.26 (n = 1112) and 0.78 ± 0.22 (n = 1692), respectively. The area under the curve (AUC) of the receiver operating characteristic (ROC) curve for low- and high-arousal data classified by ALVI1 was 0.89. The cutoff value was ALVI1 = 0.53, at which the sensitivity and specificity were 0.86 and 0.78, respectively.

8.2.3 Arousal Level Voice Index Using Sound Pressure Change Acceleration

This section introduces a different arousal level voice index from ALVI1, as described in the previous section (Shinohara et al. 2021). Consider a sound pressure level signal, that is, $x(t),\ 0 \le t \le T$. The rate of change of the sound pressure $v(t)$ at time t is given by

$$v(t)=\frac{x(t)-x(t-1)}{\Delta t} \tag{8.4}$$

The acceleration of change in sound pressure A is then defined as follows.

$$a(t)=\frac{1}{\text{mean}\left(\left|v(t+1)\right|,\left|v(t)\right|\right)}\frac{v(t+1)-v(t)}{\Delta t} \tag{8.5}$$

where mean(x, y) represents the mean of x and y and is used for normalization. In this study, the harmonic mean is used as the mean. For simplicity, we set it as $\Delta t = 1$. Equation (8.5) can then be rewritten as

$$a(t)=\frac{\left|v(t+1)\right|+\left|v(t)\right|}{2\left|v(t+1)\right|\left|v(t)\right|}\left[v(t+1)-v(t)\right] \tag{8.6}$$

We now focus on the directionality of $a(t)$. The centerline was defined as the time-averaged $\bar{x}$ of the signal.

$$\bar{x}=\frac{\sum_{t=0}^{T}x(t)}{T+1} \tag{8.7}$$

In the case of $a(t) < 0$, $a(t)$ represents downward acceleration. Therefore, when $x(t)$ is above the centerline, that is, $x(t)-\bar{x}>0$, $a(t)$ represents the acceleration toward the centerline. Conversely, when $x(t)$ is below the centerline, that is, $x(t)-\bar{x}<0$, $a(t)$ represents the acceleration away from the centerline. In contrast, in the case of $a(t) > 0$, $a(t)$ represents upward acceleration. Therefore, when $x(t)$ is above the centerline, that is, $x(t)-\bar{x}>0$, $a(t)$ represents the acceleration away from the centerline. Conversely, when $x(t)$ is below the centerline, that is, $x(t)-\bar{x}<0$, $a(t)$ represents the acceleration toward the centerline.

The voice index, where the acceleration toward the centerline is positive and the acceleration away from the centerline is negative, is referred to in this paper as arousal level voice index 2 (ALVI2) and is defined as follows:

$$\text{ALVI2}(t)=\begin{cases}-a(t) & \text{if } x(t)-\bar{x}>0\\ a(t) & \text{otherwise}\end{cases} \tag{8.8}$$

ALVI2 for a given overall speech signal is defined as the time average of ALVI2(t) as follows:

$$\text{ALVI2}=\frac{\sum_{t=1}^{T-1}\text{ALVI2}(t)}{T-1} \tag{8.9}$$

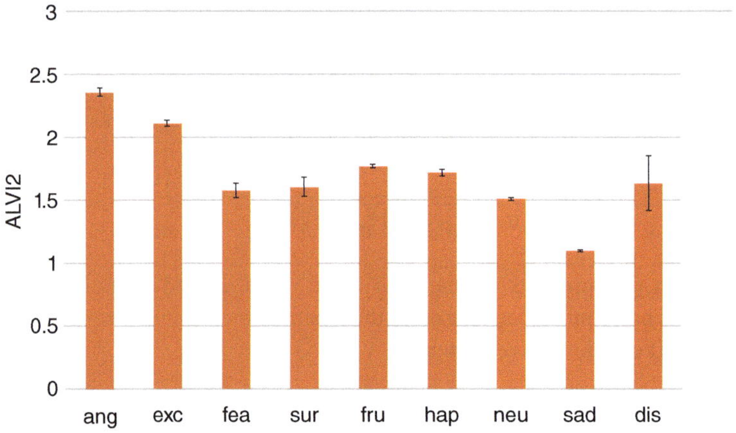

Fig. 8.5 The mean ALVI2 value for each emotion category. (Modified from Shinohara et al. 2021) *Note:* Error bars represent standard error. In addition, *ang* angry, *exc* excited, *fea* fearful, *sur* surprised, *fru* frustrated, *hap* happy, *neu* neutral, *sad* sad, and *dis* disgusted

It is clear from this definition that ALVI2 increases as the ratio of acceleration toward the center increases.

Note that, as can be seen from Eq. (8.6), ALVI2 is invariant with respect to scaling in the amplitude direction because of the normalization process used in its calculation.

We calculated ALVI2 for all 10,039 utterances in the IEMOCAP database, with a correlation coefficient of 0.52 (n = 10,039, $p < 2.2 \times 10^{-16}$) between ALVI2 and the emotional arousal level given by the raters.

Next, ALVI2 was obtained for each emotional category. Figure 8.5 shows the ALVI2 average for each category. As shown in Fig. 8.2, the emotion categories on the horizontal axis are arranged in order of the average emotional arousal given by the raters. Similar to the emotional arousal level given by the raters, ALVI2 is high for "ang" and "exc" and low for "neu" and "sad." However, as can be seen by comparing Fig. 8.5 with Fig. 8.2, the three categories of "fearful," "surprised," and "disgusted" do not match the ordinal relationship between emotional arousal and ALVI2.

"Fearful," "surprised," "frustrated," and "happy" are reversed in order in emotional arousal and ALVI2, but as Fig. 8.4 shows, there is little difference in the emotional arousal of these four categories. In other words, these four categories of emotional arousal are difficult to distinguish even for humans. The order of the "disgusted" category was significantly different from that of the emotional arousal level and ALVI2, but this may be due to the sample size being too small ($n = 2$).

Next, as with ALVI 1, we evaluated the discriminative performance of ALVI2 using low-arousal data (n = 1112, arousal mean ± standard deviation SD = 1.92 ± 0.19) with arousal levels below 2 and high-arousal data (n = 1692, arousal mean ± SD = 4.19 ± 0.28) with arousal levels above 4. The AUC for the classification of low- and high-arousal data using ALVI2 was 0.93. The cutoff value was ALVI2 = 0.90, at which both the sensitivity and specificity were 0.86.

8.3 Depression Severity Assessment by ALVI

8.3.1 Voice Data and HAM-D Scores for Patients with Depression

We collected 17 Japanese fixed-phrase speech utterances from patients with major depression attending two facilities, a clinic (H1) and a hospital (H2), to assess depression severity using ALVI1 and ALVI2. However, the 17 phrases collected at both facilities were not the same: only 10 phrases were common. Therefore, only the ten common phrases shown in Table 8.1 were included in the analysis in the evaluation.

Table 8.2 shows patient information at each facility.

To measure the severity of depression, psychiatrists scored the patients' major depression severity using the HAM-D at the time of voice recording. This resulted in 10 phrase-audio recordings paired with the HAM-D scores from 178 patients with depression.

Table 8.1 Ten canned phrases used in the analysis

Phrase	Phrase in Japanese	Purpose (meaning)
P1	I-ro-ha-ni-ho-he-to	Nonemotional (no meaning, similar to "a-b-c")
P2	Honjitsu ha seiten nari	Nonemotional (It is fine today)
P5	Mukashi aru tokoro ni	Nonemotional (Once upon a time, there lived)
P11	Garapagosu shotou	Check pronunciation (Galápagos Islands)
P12	Tsukarete guttari shiteimasu.	Emotional (I am tired/dead tired)
P13	Totemo genki desu	Emotional (I am very cheerful)
P14	Kinou ha yoku nemuremashita	Emotional (I was able to sleep well yesterday)
P15	Shokuyoku ga arimasu	Emotional (I have an appetite)
P16	Okorippoi desu	Emotional (I am irritable)
P17	Kokoroga odayaka desu	Emotional (My heart is calm)

Table 8.2 Patient information

Hospital	Sex	Number of subjects	Mean age ± SD
H1	Female	55	31.6 ± 8.6
	Male	33	32.5 ± 6.5
	Total	88	32.0 ± 7.9
H2	Female	44	62.0 ± 13.1
	Male	46	48.8 ± 13.5
	Total	90	55.2 ± 14.8

Table 8.3 Mean HAM-D scores for each group per facility

Hospital	Group	Number of subjects	Mean HAM-D score ± SD
H1	No-depression (HAM-D < 8)	10	4.8 ± 1.3
	Depression (HAM-D ≥ 8)	78	24.4 ± 8.5
	Total	88	22.2 ± 10.1
H2	No-depression (HAM-D < 8)	65	2.2 ± 2.2
	Depression (HAM-D ≥ 8)	25	15.3 ± 7.2
	Total	90	5.8 ± 7.2

Although there is much debate regarding severity classification using the HAM-D (Zimmerman et al. 2013), this study used Hashim's method and divided subjects into two groups: no-depression group with HAM-D score <8 and depression group with HAM-D score ≥8 (depression group) (Hashim et al. 2017). Table 8.3 shows the mean HAM-D scores for each group by facility.

8.3.2 Discrimination Performance of ALVI1

Table 8.4 shows the discrimination performance of using ALVI1 to classify the no-depression and depression groups. This table shows the results of the Wilcoxon rank–sum test comparing the mean of ALVI1 for each group and the AUC for each phrase when groups were discriminated using ALVI1.

H1 showed the highest discrimination performance for phrase 12, with an AUC of 0.70 (cutoff point = 0. 14; sensitivity = 0.70; specificity = 0.73). In contrast, H2 had the highest discrimination performance for phrase 5, with an AUC of 0.74 (cutoff point = 0.30, sensitivity = 0.85, specificity = 0.60).

The bottom row of Table 8.4 shows the discriminative performance when using the ALVI1 mean of all ten phrases; comparison between groups using the Wilcoxon rank–sum test showed significant differences at the 10% level for H1 and 1% level for H2. The AUC was 0.66 for H1 (cutoff point = 0.20, sensitivity = 0.60,

Table 8.4 A summary of classification performance between the no-depression and depression groups by ALVI1

	p value[a]		AUC	
Phrase	H1	H2	H1	H2
P1	3.3×10^{-1}	2.7×10^{-2}*	0.60	0.65
P2	3.0×10^{-1}	$9,2 \times 10^{-3}$**	0.60	0.68
P5	2.0×10^{-1}	**6.0×10^{-4}***	0.63	**0.74**
P11	9.6×10^{-2}*	2.9×10^{-1}	0.66	0.57
P12	**4.0×10^{-2}***	1.6×10^{-2}*	**0.70**	0.67
P13	1.7×10^{-1}	4.7×10^{-3}**	0.63	0.69
P14	$9,6 \times 10^{-2}$*	6.2×10^{-3}**	0.66	0.69
P15	$9,9 \times 10^{-2}$*	4.0×10^{-2}*	0.66	0.64
P16	1.9×10^{-1}	2.2×10^{-2}*	0.63	0.68
P17	2.8×10^{-1}	2.8×10^{-2}*	0.61	0.65
All	9.4×10^{-2}*	3.8×10^{-3}**	0.66	0.70

Note. The minimum *p* value and maximum AUC for each hospital are shown in bold. *** ($p < 0.001$), ** ($p < 0.01$), * ($p < 0.1$). [a]Wilcoxon rank–sum test

specificity = 0.78) and 0.70 for H2 (cutoff point = 0.23, sensitivity = 0.85, specificity = 0.56).

8.3.3 *Discrimination Performance of ALVI2*

Table 8.5 shows the discrimination performance of using ALVI2 to classify the no-depression and depression groups. The table shows the results of the Wilcoxon rank–sum test comparing the mean ALVI2 values for each group and the AUC for each phrase when the groups were discriminated using ALVI2.

On one hand, in H1, phrase 5 had the highest discrimination performance, with an AUC of 0.76 (cutoff point = 0.53, sensitivity = 0.90, specificity = 0.58). On the other hand, H2 had the highest discriminative performance for phrase 2, with an AUC of 0.76 (cutoff point = 0.65, sensitivity = 0.83, specificity = 0.68).

The bottom row of Table 8.5 shows the discriminative performance when using the ALVI2 mean of all ten phrases; comparison between groups using the Wilcoxon rank–sum test showed significant differences at the 1% level for both H1 and H2. The AUC was 0.76 for H1 (cutoff point = 0.62, sensitivity = 0.80, specificity = 0.73) and 0.72 for H2 (cutoff point = 0.63, sensitivity = 0.89, specificity = 0.48).

Table 8.5 A summary of classification performance between the no-depression and depression groups by ALVI2

	p value[a]		AUC	
Phrase	H1	H2	H1	H2
P1	1.9×10^{-2}*	5.6×10^{-3}**	0.73	0.69
P2	2.6×10^{-2}*	**1.5×10^{-4}*** **	0.72	**0.76**
P5	**7.3×10^{-3}** **	8.9×10^{-3}**	**0.76**	0.68
P11	8.6×10^{-3}**	5.3×10^{-3}**	0.76	0.69
P12	1.2×10^{-2}*	5.8×10^{-3}**	0.75	0.69
P13	1.7×10^{-2}*	6.6×10^{-3}**	0.73	0.69
P14	7.6×10^{-3}**	1.9×10^{-3}**	0.76	0.71
P15	1.9×10^{-2}*	1.6×10^{-2}*	0.73	0.67
P16	2.5×10^{-1}	2.4×10^{-3}**	0.61	0.71
P17	3.6×10^{-1}	5.0×10^{-2}*	0.59	0.63
All	8.9×10^{-3}**	1.6×10^{-3}**	0.76	0.72

Note. The minimum p value and maximum AUC for each hospital are shown in bold. *** ($p < 0.001$), ** ($p < 0.01$), * ($p < 0.1$). [a]Wilcoxon rank–sum test

8.4 Discussion and Conclusions

In this study, we examined the possibility of using the emotional arousal estimated from speech to detect depression. First, we examined the relationship between emotional categories and ratings of emotional arousal using voice data from IEMOCAP (Busso et al. 2008). We found that people perceived higher arousal for voices characterized by anger and excitement and lower arousal for voices characterized by neutral, sadness, and disgust.

We then developed two voice measures, ALVI1 and ALVI2, to measure emotional arousal from voice. The former focuses on the relationship between HE and ZCR, whereas the latter focuses on the acceleration of the change in sound pressure.

To evaluate the developed speech indices, low-arousal data (n = 1112) with arousal level 2 or lower and high-arousal data (n = 1692) with arousal level 4 or higher were used out of 10,039 utterances in IEMOCAP.

The AUC was 0.89, when the low- and high-arousal data were classified using ALVI1. However, when low- and high-arousal data were classified using ALVI2, the AUC was 0.93. Thus, using ALVI1 and ALVI2, low- and high-arousal speech can be discriminated with very high accuracy.

Next, we extracted ALVI1 and ALVI2 from the speech of depressed patients and investigated the relationship between these speech measures and depression severity using the HAM-D score. Data were collected at two sites: H1 and H2.

For ALVI1 in the no-depression and depression groups, the Wilcoxon rank–sum test for comparison between the groups showed significant differences at the 10% level for H1 and at the 1% level for H2.

In the case of ALVI2, the difference is significant at the 1% level for both H1 and H2.

When ALVI1 was used to classify the no-depression and depression groups separately, the AUC was 0.66 for H1 and 0.70 for H2. However, when ALVI2 was used to classify both groups, the area under the AUC was 0.76 H1 and 0.72 H2. Thus, it is suggested that the ALVI and ALVI2 could be used to discriminate between the no-depression and depression groups.

This study has several limitations. First, the arousal level voice indices (ALVI1 and ALVI2) proposed in this paper vary in value from phrase to phrase; therefore, the same phrases must be used to accurately compare healthy subjects and patients with depression. In the future, it will be necessary to improve the proposed indices such that they can be applied to free speech.

Second, the arousal level used in the development of the proposed indices was a rating value given by the annotator and was not based on the subject's own evaluation. Therefore, it is necessary to investigate the relationship between the proposed index and the subject's self-evaluation and physiological index in the future.

Third, with respect to the data used in this study, the sample size for each group was small. We collected voices from two sites, but the age groups and distribution of the HAM-D scores were quite different. The mean age of the patients was higher in the H2 group than in the H1 group. In contrast, the mean HAM-D score was higher for the H1. The reasons for these differences are as follows: H1 was located in central Tokyo, and most outpatients were young office workers who commuted to the city center. In contrast, H2 is located in the suburbs and has many elderly outpatients living in the area. In addition, H2 was a university hospital, and many patients had already received treatment at another hospital. In the future, the findings of this study should be validated using a larger dataset collected in the same setting.

Fourth, the current study failed to address the issue of specificity. Other illnesses besides depression are associated with arousal, and low arousal does not necessarily indicate high severity of depression. For example, apathy may be associated with neurodegenerative diseases such as Alzheimer's disease (AD), frontotemporal dementia (FTD), Parkinson's disease, dementia with Lewy bodies, and other neurological diseases and may overlap with other neuropsychiatric syndromes such as depression. Disruptions in the same brain networks involved in arousal, threat response, and reward processing are also associated with apathy in AD and FTD (Huey et al. 2017). In the future, new indices that can differentiate major depression from the aforementioned disorders should be developed.

References

American Psychiatric Association (2000) Steering Committee on Practice Guidelines, American Psychiatric Association, Practice Guidelines for the Treatment of Psychiatric Disorders: Compendium 2000. American Psychiatric Association, Arlington

Bachu R, Kopparthi S, Adapa B, Barkana B (2010) Voiced/unvoiced decision for speech signals based on zero-crossing rate and energy. In: Elleithy K (ed) Advanced techniques in computing sciences and software engineering. Springer, Dordrecht, pp 279–282

Benning SD, Ait Oumeziane B (2017) Reduced positive emotion and underarousal are uniquely associated with subclinical depression symptoms: evidence from psychophysiology, self-report, and symptom clusters. Psychophysiology 54(7):1010–1030. https://doi.org/10.1111/psyp.12853

Bone D, Lee CC, Narayanan S (2014) Robust unsupervised arousal rating: a rule-based framework with knowledge-inspired vocal features. IEEE Trans Affect Comput 5(2):201–213. https://doi.org/10.1109/TAFFC.2014.2326393

Busso C, Bulut M, Lee C, Kazemzadeh A, Mower E, Kim S, Chang JN, Lee S, Narayanan SS (2008) IEMOCAP: interactive emotional dyadic motion capture database. Lang Resour Eval 42:335

Cronbach L (1951) Coefficient alpha and the internal structure of tests. Psychometrika 16:297–334

Ekman P, Friesen W (1971) Constants across cultures in the face and emotion. J Pers Soc Psychol 17(2):124–129

Eom C, Choi S, Oh G, Jung WS (2008) Hurst exponent and prediction based on weak-form ecient market hypothesis of stock markets. Physica A 387:4630–4636

Fleiss J (1981) Statistical methods for rates and proportions. Wiley

Hashim NW, Wilkes M, Salomon R, Meggs J, France DJ (2017) Evaluation of voice acoustics as predictors of clinical depression scores. J Voice 31:256.e1–256.e6

Huey ED, Lee S, Cheran G, Grafman J Devanand DP (2017) Brain regions involved in arousal and reward processing are associated with apathy in Alzheimer's disease and frontotemporal dementia. J Alzheimers Dis 55(2), 551-558; https://doi.org/10.3233/JAD-160107.

Jalil M, Butt FA, Malik A (2013) Short-time energy, magnitude, zero-crossing rate and autocorrelation measurement for discriminating voiced and unvoiced segments of speech signals. In: Proceedings of the 2013 international conference on technological advances in electrical, electronics and computer engineering (TAEECE), Konya, Turkey, 9–11 May 2013, pp 208–212

Kazi MH, Ekramul H, Khademul IMA (2017) Method for voiced/unvoiced classification of noisy speech by analyzing time-domain features of spectrogram image. Sci J Circuits Syst Signal Process 6:11–17

Moratti S, Rubio G, Campo P, Keil A, Ortiz T (2008) Hypofunction of right temporoparietal cortex during emotional arousal in depression. Arch Gen Psychiatry 65:532–541

Schmidt, Janse E, Scharenborg O (2016) Perception of emotion in conversational speech by younger and older listeners. Front Psychol 7:781

Schmidt FM, Sander C, Dietz ME, Nowak C, Schröder T, Mergl R, Schönknecht P, Himmerich H, Hegerl U (2017) Brain arousal regulation as response predictor for antidepressant therapy in major depression. Sci Rep 7:45187. https://doi.org/10.1038/srep45187

Shinohara S, Toda H, Nakamura M, Omiya Y, Higuchi M, Takano T, Saito T, Tanichi M, Boku S, Mitsuyoshi S, So M, Yoshino A, Tokuno S (2020) Evaluation of the severity of major depression using a voice index for emotional arousal. Sensors (Basel) 20(18):5041

Shinohara S, Toda H, Nakamura M et al (2021) Evaluation of emotional arousal level and depression severity using voice-derived sound pressure change acceleration. Sci Rep 11:13615

Sobin C, Sackeim HA (1997) Psychomotor symptoms of depression. Am J Psychiatry 154(1):4–17. https://doi.org/10.1176/ajp.154.1.4

Zimmerman M, Martinez JH, Young D, Chelminski I, Dalrymple K (2013) Severity classification on the Hamilton Depression Rating Scale. J Affect Disord 150(2):384–388. https://doi.org/10.1016/j.jad.2013.04.028. Epub 2013 Jun 4

Chapter 9
Depression: Machine Learning

Yasuhiro Omiya

In this study, the development of an algorithm for estimating depression based on machine learning combined with acoustic features analyzed from speech is presented (Omiya et al. 2018, 2019).

In this study, the voices of patients with major depressive disorder (MDD) were recorded with their consent in a clinical examination room. The Hamilton Depression Rating Scale (HAM-D) was used by a psychiatrist to screen for depression, and the M.I.N.I-International Neuropsychiatric Interview (M.I.N.I.) was used to exclude serious physical disorders or organic brain disorders (Sheehan et al. 1998). For the recordings, native language-independent sustained vowels were selected, and the participants' voices were recorded as they uttered the vowels /Ah/, /Eh/, and /Uh/ for approximately 3 s each. The recording was made using a portable recorder R-26 (Roland, Japan) and a pin microphone ME-52W (OLYMPUS, Japan) in PCM format at 24 bit/96 kHz. After the second visit, we collected the subjects' voices and conducted the HAM-D at each visit to observe the progress of the patient's recovery. In many cases, as the patients were treated by a doctor, their symptoms improved. On the other hand, as some patients did not revisit the hospital when their condition improved, their voices could not be recorded. Data were collected from 28 participants, and the total number of data points was 42, as shown in Table 9.1.

For the analysis of acoustic features from the collected participant speech, 6552 acoustic features were calculated using the openSMILE software (Eyben et al. 2010). The acoustic features were calculated using the following procedure.

- (a) Physical feature was calculated on the basis of a frame unit or 56 similar feature types.
- (b) Three processing contents (moving average and time change) in the time direction concerning (a).

Y. Omiya (✉)
Research and Development Department, PST Inc., Yokohama, Kanagawa, Japan
e-mail: omiya@medical-pst.com

S. Tokuno, H. Nakamura (eds.), *Voice Biomarkers*,
https://doi.org/10.1007/978-981-96-3109-4_9

Table 9.1 Collected participant's information

	Number of recordings			Age			HAM-D score	
Gender	Once	Twice	3 times	Mean ± S.D.	t-test	Number of data	Mean ± S.D.	t-test
Male	5	5	1	32.5 ± 5.9	n.s.	20	23.3 ± 11.1	n.s.
Female	10	7	0	32.2 ± 8.6		22	25.0 ± 9.3	

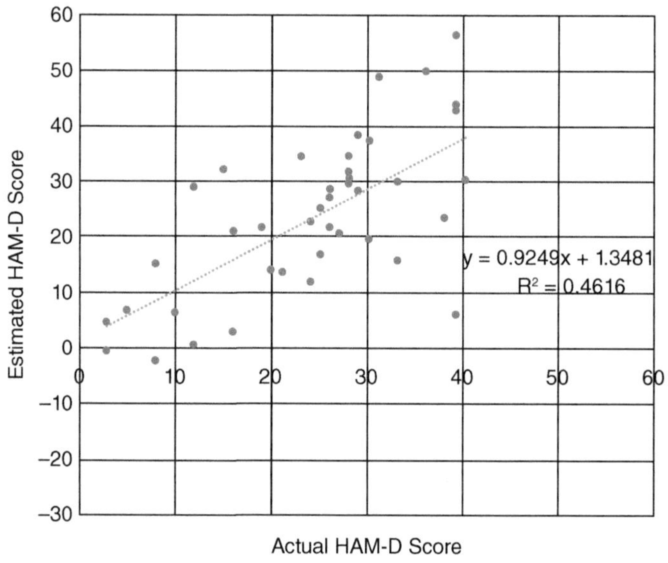

Fig. 9.1 Scatterplot for the "Estimated HAM-D Score" versus the "Actual HAM-D Score" based on the acoustic features of /Ah/

– (c) After process (b) is performed on (a), statistical quantities of 39 types.

Then, for machine learning, feature selection was performed using Weka (Hall et al. 2009), a data mining tool provided by the University of Waikato, with the "CfsSubsetEval" and "BestFirst" settings. Next, a HAM-D score estimation algorithm was created using the sequential minimal optimization method implemented in Weka with ten-fold cross-validation. In the analysis, the correlation coefficient between the "Actual HAM-D Score" and the "Estimated HAM-D Score" was evaluated according to generated algorithm.

Figures 9.1, 9.2, and 9.3 show the scatterplots of the "Estimated HAM-D Score" and the "Actual HAM-D Score" from an algorithm generated based on machine learning combining acoustic features analyzed from the speech of /Ah/, /Eh/ and /Uh/.

The results show that the correlation coefficients between the estimated and actual HAM-D scores, based on an algorithm created by machine learning combining acoustic features analyzed from speech, were 0.68, 0.83, and 0.68, respectively. Among them, the correlation coefficient for /Eh/ was very high at approximately

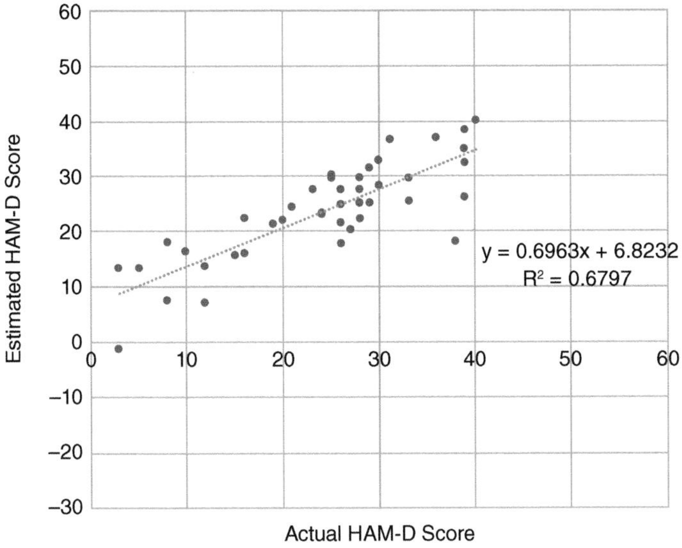

Fig. 9.2 Scatterplot for the "Estimated HAM-D Score" versus the "Actual HAM-D Score" based on the acoustic features of /Eh/

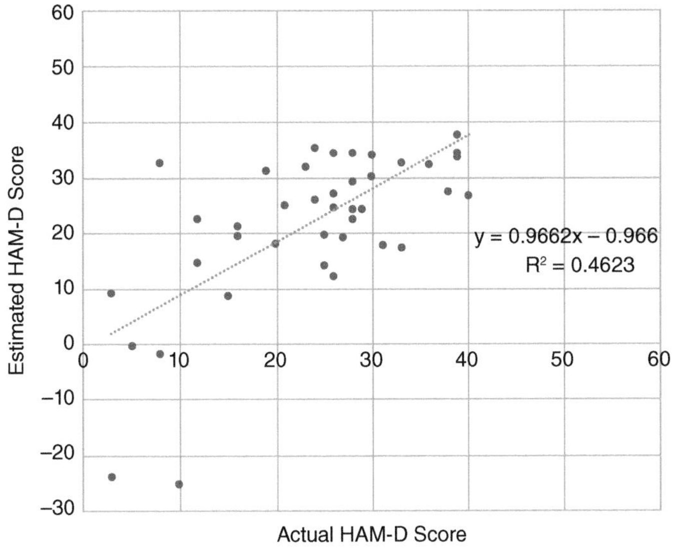

Fig. 9.3 Scatterplot for the "Estimated HAM-D Score" versus the "Actual HAM-D Score" based on the acoustic features of /Uh/

0.83, and for /Ah/ and /Uh/, the correlation coefficient was more than 0.65, suggesting that the estimated HAM-D score based on the acoustic features of sustained vowels /Ah/, /Eh/, and /Uh/ is effective for estimating depressive states and can be used to estimate depressive symptoms through speech.

The algorithm performance was then evaluated to check if the subjects' voices could serve as a parameter to identify those with depressive mental health conditions, as indicated by a HAM-D score of 17 or higher, the cut-off point for "exhibiting moderate depression," as discussed by Zimmerman et al. (2013).

Figures 9.4, 9.5, and 9.6 show the receiver operating characteristic (ROC) curves of the discrimination performance based on the HAM-D scores from the algorithm created based on machine learning by combining the acoustic features analyzed from the /Ah/, /Eh/, and /Uh/ speech.

The results show that the "discrimination performance based on HAM-D Scores" using the "Estimated HAM-D Scores" with acoustic features of /Ah/, /Eh/ and /Uh/ has an area under the ROC curve (AUC) value of 0.84, 0.98 and 0.87. These results indicate that the generated algorithm works correctly in estimating the severity of the HAM-D score using the acoustic features of sustained vowels, suggesting that it is effective in estimating the mental health status based on speech.

A scatterplot of the "average of the Estimated HAM-D Score based on the acoustic features of the three sustained vowels /Ah/, /Eh/ and /Uh/" and the "Actual HAM-D Score" is shown in Fig. 9.7, and an ROC curve showing the "discrimination performance based on the HAM-D Score" using the average of the "Estimated HAM-D Scores" of the three sustained vowels is also shown in Fig. 9.8.

The results show that the correlation coefficient between the "Estimated HAM-D Score" and the "Actual HAM-D Score" for the three combined sustained vowels /Ah/, /Eh/, and /Uh/ is 0.833, and the area under the ROC curve (AUC) value was 0.95. These results suggest that a combination of the three sustained vowels is effective in estimating the severity of the HAM-D score and in estimating persons with a depressed mental state.

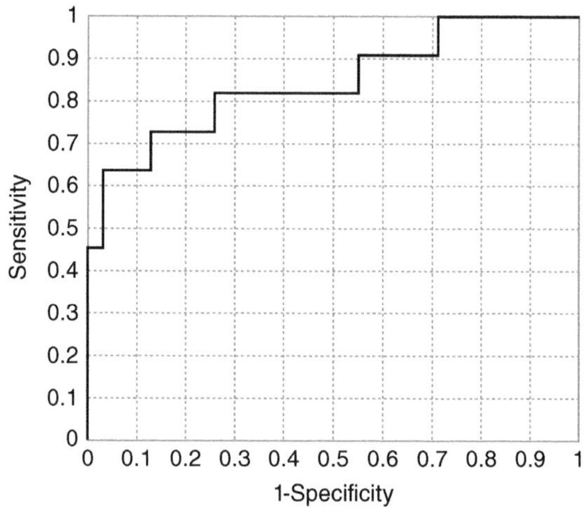

Fig. 9.4 ROC curve of the "Estimated HAM-D Score" using the acoustic features of /Ah/

Fig. 9.5 ROC curve of the "Estimated HAM-D Score" using the acoustic features of /Eh/

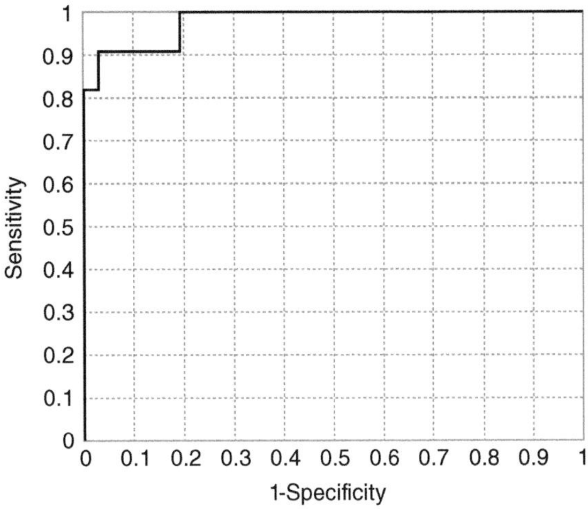

Fig. 9.6 ROC curve of the "Estimated HAM-D Score" using the acoustic features of /Uh/

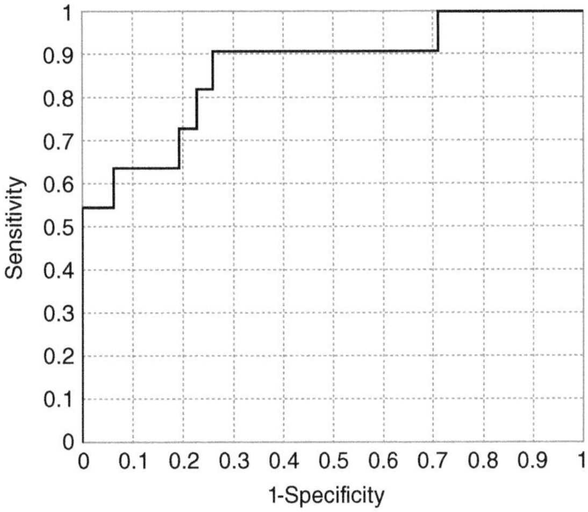

In this study, an algorithm to "estimate HAM-D scores using the acoustic features of three language-independent sustained vowels /Ah/, /Eh/, and /Uh/ was developed. The "Estimated HAM-D Score" from the algorithm created based on machine learning combined with acoustic features analyzed from speech was then compared and validated with the "Actual HAM-D Score." The results suggest that the developed algorithm works correctly in estimating the severity of the HAM-D score, which indicates depression and can be used to estimate depressive mental states based on speech.

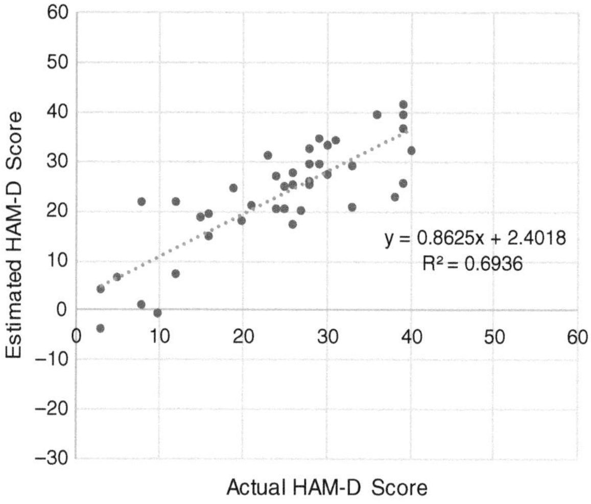

Fig. 9.7 Scatterplot of the "Estimated HAM-D Score" versus the "Actual HAM-D Score" based on the acoustic features of /Ah/, /Eh/, and /Uh/ by calculating the average value

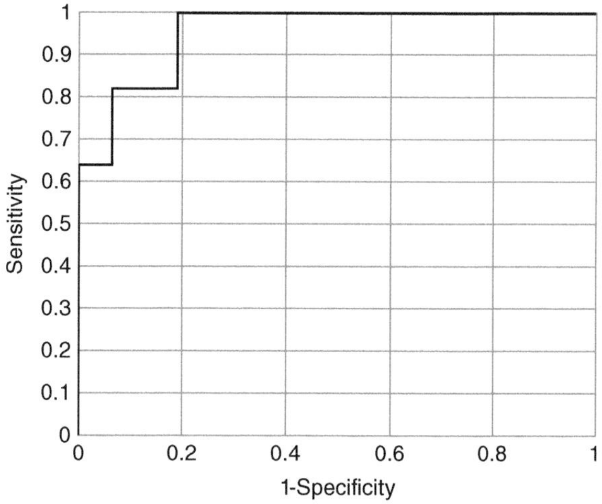

Fig. 9.8 ROC curve of the "Estimated HAM-D Score" using the acoustic features of /Ah/, /Eh/, and /Uh/ by calculating the average value

References

Eyben F, Wllmer M, Schuller B (2010) Opensmile: the Munich versatile and fast open-source audio feature extractor. In: Bimbo AD, Chang SF, Smeulders AWM (eds) ACM multimedia, pp 1459–1462

Hall M et al (2009) The WEKA data mining software: an update. ACM SIGKDD Explorations Newsl 11(1):10–18

Omiya Y, Takano T, Uraguchi T, Higuchi M, Shinohara S, Nakamura M, Mitsuyoshi S, So M, Tokuno S (2018) Estimating depressive status from voice. In: The 2018 IEEE international conference on bioinformatics and biomedicine (BIBM2018), Madrid, 3–6 December 2018

Omiya Y, Takano T, Uraguchi T, Nakamura M, Higuchi M, Shinohara S, Mitsuyoshi S, So M, Tokuno S (2019) An attempt to estimate depressive status from voice. Pervasive Computing

Paradigms for Mental Health (MindCare 2019). Lecture notes of the institute for computer sciences, social informatics and telecommunications engineering, vol 288, pp 168–175
Sheehan DV, Lecrubier Y, Sheehan KH, Amorim P, Janavs J, Weiller E, Hergueta T, Baker R, Dunbar GC (1998) The Mini-International Neuropsychiatric Interview (M.I.N.I): the development and validation of a structured diagnostic psychiatric interview for DSM-IV and ICD-10. J Clin Psychiatry 59(Suppl 20):22–33
Zimmerman M, Martinez JH, Young D, Chelminski I, Dalrymple K (2013) Severity classification on the Hamilton Depression Rating Scale. Epub 150(2):384–388

Chapter 10
Depression: Logistic Regression

Masakazu Higuchi

10.1 Detection of Depression in the Elderly

In recent years, the world's population has been aging (United Nations Population Division 2002). Elderly people often develop depression due to decline in physical functions, health concerns, bereavement of friends, and loneliness, and it is one of the most common diseases among the elderly along with dementia (Beekman et al. 1999). We proposed a voice evaluation index based on logistic regression to detect depression in the elderly that replaces vitality and mental activity by combining the emotional components of the voice (Higuchi et al. 2017, 2018a).

These studies included 35 elderly people aged 65 years or older who were using the Mind Monitoring System (MIMOSYS) (Shinohara et al. 2021) smartphone application during the first half of the period when the smartphone application was open to the public in a prospective study (Higuchi et al. 2020). The users completed the questionnaire of Beck Depression Inventory (BDI) (Beck et al. 1961) on their smartphones every 3 months from the start of application use. Voice samples were acquired from calls made within 2 weeks of the BDI questionnaire. We judged that data within 2 weeks of the BDI questionnaire were valid because the American Psychiatric Association diagnostic criteria for depression state that depression lasts for at least 2 weeks (American Psychiatric Association 2000). Some users completed the BDI questionnaire multiple times. Among the aforementioned 35 users, 33 made calls within 2 weeks of the BDI questionnaire, and 41 valid BDI scores were obtained. The total number of valid voices was 672. Data were grouped according to the BDI score evaluation criteria. These criteria have been reported to screen patients with depression with high accuracy (Beck et al. 1996). The users

M. Higuchi (✉)
Department of Bioengineering, Graduate School of Engineering, The University of Tokyo, Bunkyo-ku, Tokyo, Japan
e-mail: higuchi@bioeng.t.u-tokyo.ac.jp

S. Tokuno, H. Nakamura (eds.), *Voice Biomarkers*,
https://doi.org/10.1007/978-981-96-3109-4_10

were classified into two groups: one group included users with a BDI score of 17 or higher and requiring a doctor's diagnosis (clinical depression), and the other group included users with a BDI score of less than 17 and did not require a doctor's diagnosis (normal). The valid voices of users in each group were analyzed. The numbers of users in the clinical depression and normal groups were 3 and 30, respectively. The users that completed the BDI questionnaire multiple times and were classified into the clinical depression group based on their first BDI score also had a BDI score of 17 or higher for the second and subsequent BDI scores. Similarly, users that were classified into the normal group based on their first BDI score also had a BDI score of less than 17 on the second and subsequent BDI scores. This implies that there was no overlap of users between the two groups. There were 50 and 622 voice data points in the clinical depression and control groups, respectively.

Logistic regression analysis (Agresti 2012) was applied to the emotional components (calmness, anger, joy, sorrow, and excitement) as explanatory variables calculated by the sensibility technology (ST) (Mitsuyoshi et al. 2006) of MIMOSYS from the voice data of the two groups. Hence, we obtained the depression evaluation index (DEI), which consists of anger, joy, sorrow, and excitement components. By applying the emotional components contained in voice to the DEI, we can predict the probability that the voice is classified as a clinical depression group. Figure 10.1 shows the distribution of the predicted values calculated using the DEI from the voice data belonging to each group. A significant difference ($p < 0.01$) was confirmed using a t-test between the mean predicted values of the two groups. The receiver operating characteristic (ROC) curve for DEI is shown in Fig. 10.2. For comparison with MIMOSYS, the ROC curve for vitality is shown. The area under the curve (AUC) of DEI was 0.761 and that of vitality was 0.635. The best cut-off

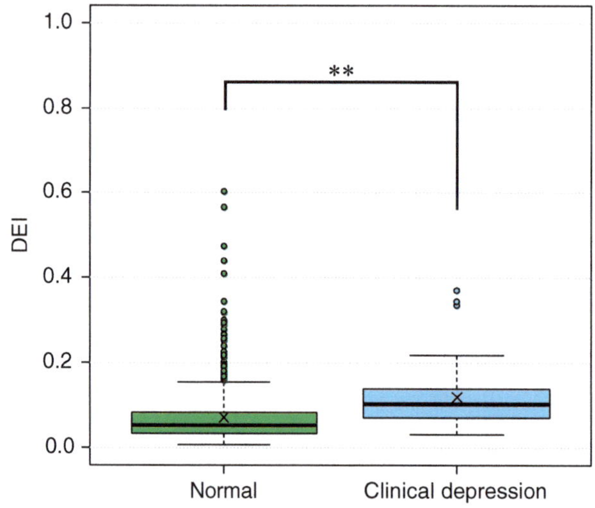

Fig. 10.1 Distribution of DEI predictions for normal and clinical depression groups ($**\,p < 0.01$). (Modified from Higuchi et al. 2017)

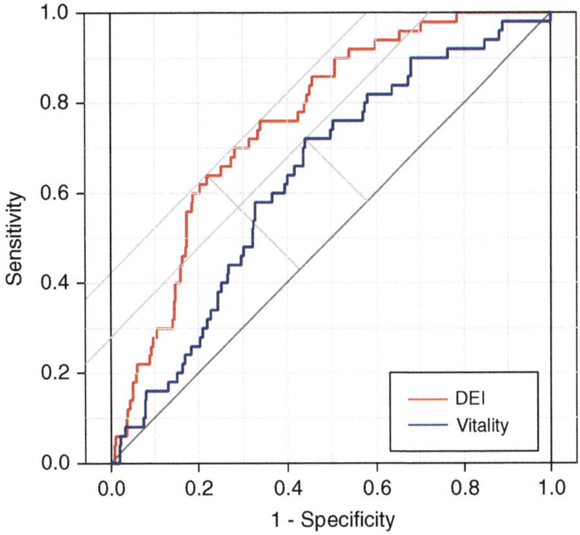

Fig. 10.2 ROC curves for DEI and vitality of MIMOSYS. (Modified from Higuchi et al. 2017)

Table 10.1 Confusion matrix for the best cut-off value of DEI

		BDI	
		Normal (BDI < 17)	Clinical depression (BDI ≥ 17)
DEI	Low (< 0.0891)	485	18
	High (≥ 0.0891)	136	32

value for the DEI was 0.0891, and the sensitivity and specificity at the cut-off were 0.640 and 0.781, respectively. The confusion matrix for the cut-off values is presented in Table 10.1. Although the performance of the DEI, as a classifier, is not good, it showed a higher classification performance than the vitality of MIMOSYS, suggesting that the DEI can be effective in screening elderly patients with depression.

In addition to the emotional components, attribute information (gender, age, and history of current illness) was added to the explanatory variables, and a logistic regression analysis was applied. Gender was a qualitative variable and converted into a dummy variable. The history of current illness was defined as the number of illnesses suffered from at the time users responded to the initial questionnaire when they were registered using MIMOSYS. Hence, based on the analysis, another depression evaluation index with attribute (DEIA), composed of variables excluding the calmness component, was obtained. Figure 10.3 shows the distribution of the predicted values that are calculated using DEIA for each group. A significant difference ($p < 0.01$) was confirmed using a t-test between the mean predicted values of the two groups. The ROC curve for DEIA is shown in Fig. 10.4. For comparison, the ROC curves for the DEI, which consists of only emotional components, and vitality are also shown. The AUC under the ROC curve for DEIA was 0.93. The best cut-off value for DEIA was 0.11, and the sensitivity and specificity at the cut-off

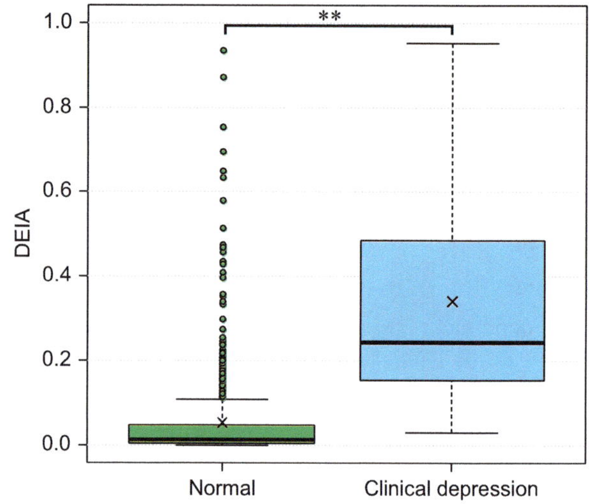

Fig. 10.3 Distribution of DEIA predictions for normal and clinical depression groups ($**p < 0.01$). (Modified from Higuchi et al. 2018a)

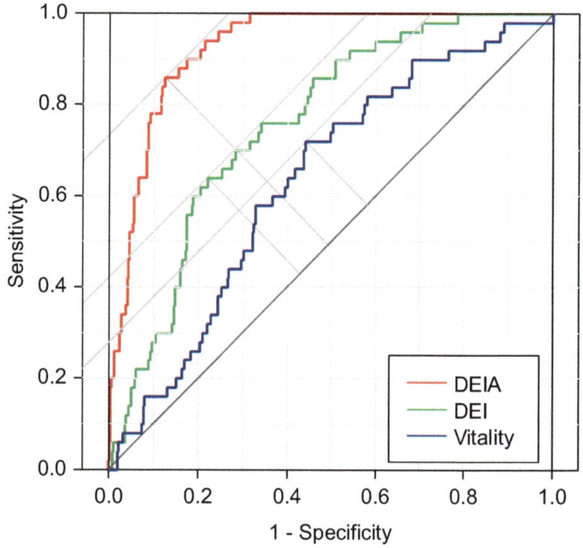

Fig. 10.4 ROC curves for DEIA, DEI, and vitality of MIMOSYS. (Modified from Higuchi et al. 2018a)

were 0.86 and 0.87, respectively. The confusion matrix for the cut-off values is presented in Table 10.2. The performance of DEIA, as a classifier, showed high values, and the performance was significantly improved when compared with that of DEI.

Table 10.2 Confusion matrix for the best cut-off value of DEIA

		BDI	
		Normal (BDI < 17)	Clinical depression (BDI ≥ 17)
DEIA	Low (<0.11)	544	7
	High (≥0.11)	78	43

10.2 Detection of Depression in Younger and Older Adults

The depression evaluation indices DEI and DEIA for the elderly were analyzed on an unspecified number of subjects using MIMOSYS, and the BDI questionnaire and initial questionnaire were conducted on smartphones. Hence, the reliability of the information was problematic to a certain extent. Therefore, in collaboration with psychiatrists, we recruited patients who were attending a hospital for the treatment of major depressive disorder and proposed a voice evaluation index to discriminate depression from their voices as an alternative to vitality and mental activity (Higuchi et al. 2018b).

In this study, we included patients diagnosed with major depressive disorder using the Mini-International Neuropsychiatric Interview (M.I.N.I.) (Sheehan et al. 1998). The normal subjects were healthy individuals who were leading their daily lives without any problems. There were 46 patients with major depressive disorder (34 males and 12 females) and 37 healthy subjects (22 males and 15 females). The mean age was 48.4 ± 11.6 (M ± SD) years. Voice recordings were acquired in hospital examination rooms, and the participants were asked to read out fixed Japanese phrases. A portable recorder R-26 (Roland, Japan) was used for voice recording. The voice was recorded using a 24 bit resolution with a sampling frequency of 96 kHz. The voices were converted to 16 bit and 11 kHz format according to MIMOSYS specifications and were analyzed via MIMOSYS to calculate the emotional components of the voices.

By applying regularized logistic regression analysis (Friedman et al. 2010) using emotional components as explanatory variables, we obtained separate depression evaluation indices for males and females. The index for males consisted of components of calmness and joy, and that for females consisted of components of joy and excitement. Figure 10.5 shows the ROC curves for male and female indices and confusion matrices for the best cut-off values. The AUCs under the ROC curves for male and female indices was 0.85 and 0.82, respectively. The sensitivity and specificity at the best cut-off values were 0.68 and 0.95 for males and 0.83 and 0.73 for females, respectively. Although the sensitivity of the male index was not high, the results suggest that these indices can be effective for screening patients with depression. Additionally, the emotional components selected for the derivation of the indices differed between males and females, suggesting that men and women potentially express their emotions in different ways.

During the course of research, it became clear that not only depression but also other diseases affect the expression of emotions, and it is difficult to distinguish

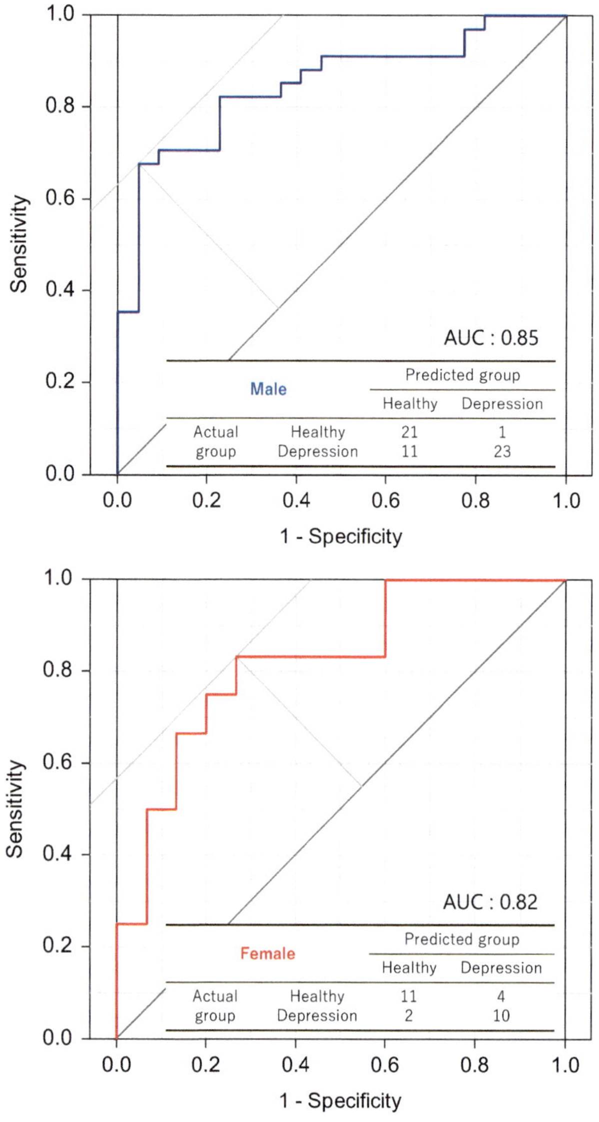

Fig. 10.5 ROC curves for male and female depression evaluation indices and confusion matrices for their best cut-off values

whether changes in emotional components are due to depression or other diseases. Therefore, we attempted an exploratory approach to directly detect depression using a combination of audio features without emotional components. We proposed a new voice evaluation index that discriminates between healthy subjects and patients with major depressive disorder using logistic regression analysis combined with principal component analysis (Higuchi et al. 2022).

In this study, we included 177 patients who were attending hospitals for treatment of major depressive disorder. Patients were diagnosed using the Mini-International Neuropsychiatric Interview (M.I.N.I.) (Sheehan et al. 1998). The severity of depression was assessed by physicians using the Hamilton Depression Rating Scale (HDRS) (Hamilton 1960). According to the evaluation criteria reported in a previous study (Riedel et al. 2010), patients with an HDRS score of less than 8 points were treated as remission, and they were excluded from the analysis. Ultimately, the study included 102 patients with major depressive disorder who had an HDRS score of ≥8. The healthy participants included 129 healthy individuals who were leading their daily lives without any problems. Voice recordings of the patients were acquired in hospital examination rooms, and those of healthy subjects were acquired in hospital examination rooms or in a soundproof booth. The voice recordings were of fixed Japanese phrases that were read aloud. A portable recorder, R-26 (Roland, Japan), was used for the voice recordings. The recording was conducted at a resolution of 24 bit and sampling frequency of 96 kHz. A free software, openSMILE version 2.3 (Eyben et al. 2010), was used to extract features from voices. OpenSMILE provides a set of scripts to automatically extract various feature sets from voice data, and we used the feature set (the large openSMILE emotion feature set) used in emotion recognition. From a single voice, we extracted 6552 (56 × 3 × 39) audio features, which were computed as follows:

Fifty-six types of acoustic/physical quantities were calculated at the frame level as low-level descriptors: fast Fourier transform (FFT), MFCCs, voiced speech probability, zero-crossing rate, signal energy, F0, etc.

Three types of temporal statistics were derived from these descriptors at the frame level: moving average, first-order change over time (delta), and second-order change over time (delta-delta).

Thirty-nine types of statistical functionals were calculated at the file (phrase) level from frame-level values: mean, maximum, minimum, centroid, quartiles, variance, kurtosis, skewness, etc.

Before learning to use the aforementioned audio features as explanatory variables, features that were effective for discrimination were selected in advance because excessive number of explanatory variables can lead to overlearning. The discriminative performance of the depressed and healthy groups for each feature was calculated using the AUC of the ROC curve, and features with an AUC greater than a certain threshold were selected. Given that some of the selected features are essentially similar to each other, principal component analysis was applied to aggregate the features with similar characteristics into several principal components. Then, regularized logistic regression analysis was applied using the obtained principal components as explanatory variables. A total of 115 healthy subjects and 77 patients with major depressive disorder were selected as training data, and the remaining 14 healthy subjects and 25 patients with major depressive disorder were selected as testing data to evaluate the obtained discriminant index.

One hundred eighty-seven features were selected as effective features for discrimination, and these features were aggregated into three principal components with a cumulative contribution rate of up to 80%. The Major Depression

Table 10.3 Discrimination result of training data

		Predicted group	
		Healthy group	Depressed group
Actual group	Healthy group	103	12
	Depressed group	5	72

Discrimination Index (MDDI) was obtained as a logistic function of the linear sum of the principal components and their corresponding regression coefficients. Table 10.3 shows the confusion matrix when the training data were discriminated between healthy subjects and patients using the best MDDI cut-off value derived from the training data. The sensitivity, specificity, and accuracy were 0.935, 0.896, and 0.911, respectively. Figure 10.6 shows the discrimination performance of MDDI for the training data as an ROC curve. The AUC was 0.97. Table 10.4 shows the confusion matrix when the testing data are discriminated between healthy subjects and patients using the best MDDI cut-off value for the training data. The sensitivity, specificity, and accuracy were 0.800, 0.786, and 0.795, respectively. The discrimination performance of the MDDI for training data was approximately 0.9 for sensitivity, specificity, and accuracy rate, and thereby, MDDI can be considered as a highly accurate index. Therefore, it was considered that there was a large difference between the voices of healthy subjects and those of patients with major depressive disorder. Hence, a discriminant index that appropriately captures this difference was obtained. The discrimination performance of the MDDI for testing data was approximately 0.8 in terms of sensitivity, specificity, and accuracy rate, indicating that overlearning did not occur. Therefore, the discriminant index obtained in this study can be considered as a new index for detecting major depressive disorders.

10.3 Conclusion

We proposed an emotion-based voice evaluation index as an alternative to MIMOSYS using logistic regression analysis.

First, we classified elderly individuals aged 65 years or older into two groups, a group with suspected depression and another group with no depression. Then, based on their scores on the BDI questionnaire, we conducted a logistic regression analysis using the emotional components calculated via ST as explanatory variables from voice calls within 2 weeks after the BDI questionnaire. Consequently, an index with higher discrimination accuracy than that of MIMOSYS was obtained. Furthermore, when logistic regression analysis was conducted using the subjects' attribute information as explanatory variables in addition to the emotional components, an index with higher discriminant accuracy than the index obtained from emotion alone was obtained. However, the reliability of the subjects' attributes and BDI questionnaire scores was low.

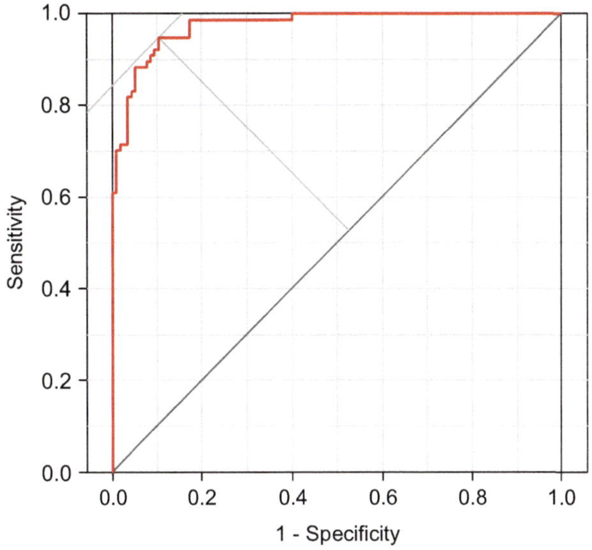

Fig. 10.6 ROC curve for MDDI values from training data. (Cited from Higuchi et al. 2022)

Table 10.4 Discrimination result of testing data

		Predicted group	
		Healthy group	Depressed group
Actual group	Healthy group	11	3
	Depressed group	5	20

Next, regularized logistic regression analysis, using the emotional components calculated via ST from voice samples of fixed Japanese phrases as explanatory variables, was conducted on subjects diagnosed with major depressive disorder by psychiatrists and healthy subjects, whose reliability was assured. Furthermore, indices with relatively high discrimination accuracy were obtained for each gender. These indices consist of different emotional components for males and females, suggesting that males and females potentially express emotions in different ways.

During the course of the study, it became clear that illnesses other than depression also affect the expression of emotions, and it is difficult to determine whether changes in emotional components are due to depression or other illnesses. Therefore, we proposed an index to detect depression by directly combining audio features without emotional components. We performed principal component analysis on the audio features calculated via openSMILE from voice samples of reading of fixed Japanese phrases in groups of normal subjects and patients with major depressive disorder. Furthermore, we applied regularized logistic regression analysis to obtained principal components. A discriminant index showing an accuracy rate of 0.9 or more for training data and an accuracy rate of approximately 0.8 for testing data was obtained. Therefore, it is suggested that the obtained discriminant index can be considered as a new index for detecting major depressive disorder with high accuracy and independent of training data.

References

Agresti A (2012) Categorical data analysis, 3rd edn. Wiley-Interscience, New York

American Psychiatric Association (2000) Diagnostic and statistical manual of mental disorders, 4th edn, Text revision. American Psychiatric Publications Inc., New York

Beck AT, Ward CH, Mendelson M, Mock J, Erbaugh J (1961) An inventory for measuring depression. Arch Gen Psychiatry 4(6):561–571

Beck AT, Steer RA, Brown GK (1996) Manual for the beck depression inventory (BDI-II), 2nd edn. Psychological Corporation, San Antonio

Beekman AT, Copeland JR, Prince MJ (1999) Review of community prevalence of depression in later life. Br J Psychiatry 174(4):307–311

Eyben F, Wöllmer M, Schuller B (2010) openSMILE—The Munich Versatile and fast open-source audio feature extractor. In: Proceedings of the 18th ACM international conference on Multimedia, Firenze, 25–29 October 2010, pp 1459–1462

Friedman J, Hastie T, Tibshirani R (2010) Regularization paths for generalized linear models via coordinate descent. J Stat Softw 33(1):1–22

Hamilton M (1960) A rating scale for depression. J Neurol Neurosurg Psychiatry 23:56–62

Higuchi M, Shinohara S, Nakamura M, Omiya Hagiwara N, Mitsuyoshi S, Tokuno S (2017) Study on depression evaluation indicator in the elderly using sensibility technology. In: Proceedings of the 3rd international conference on information and communication technologies for ageing well and e-health (ICT4AWE 2017), Porto, 28–29 April 2017: SciTePress, Portugal, pp 70–77

Higuchi M, Shinohara S, Nakamura M, Omiya Y, Hagiwara N, Takano T, Mitsuyoshi S, Tokuno S (2018a) Study on indicators for depression in the elderly using voice and attribute information. Commun Comput Inf Sci 869:127–146

Higuchi M, Shinohara S, Nakamura M, Omiya Y, Hagiwara N, Takano T, Toda H, Saito T, Terashi H, Mitoma H, Mitsuyoshi S, Tokuno S (2018b) Voice-based emotion model for identifying major depression. In: Abstracts of the 40th international engineering in medicine and biology conference (EMBC2018), Hawaii, 17–21 July 2018

Higuchi M, Nakamura M, Shinohara S, Omiya Y, Takano T, Mitsuyoshi S, Tokuno S (2020) Effectiveness of a voice-based mental health evaluation system for mobile devices: prospective study. JMIR Form Res 4(7):e16455

Higuchi M, Nakamura M, Shinohara S, Mitsuyoshi S, Omiya Y, Takano T, Mizuguchi D, Sonota N, Toda H, Saito T, So M, Takayama E, Terashi H, Mitsuyoshi S, Tokuno S (2022) Detection of major depressive disorder based on a combination of voice features: an exploratory approach. Int J Environ Res Public Health 19(18):11397

Mitsuyoshi S, Ren F, Tanaka Y, Kuroiwa S (2006) Non-verbal voice emotion analysis system. Int J Innov Comput Inf Control 2(4):819–830

Riedel M, Möller HJ, Obermeier M, Schennach-Wolff R, Bauer M, Adli M, Kronmüller K, Nickel T, Brieger P, Laux G, Bender W, Heuser I, Zeiler J, Gaebel W, Seemüller F (2010) Response and remission criteria in major depression—a validation of current practice. J Psychiatr Res 44(15):1063–1068

Sheehan DV, Lecrubier Y, Sheehan KH, Amorim P, Janavs J, Weiller E, Her-gueta T, Baker R, Dunbar GC (1998) The Mini-International Neuropsychiatric Interview (M.I.N.I): the development and validation of a structured diagnostic psychiatric interview for DSM-IV and ICD-10. J Clin Psychiatry 59(Suppl 20):22–33

Shinohara S, Nakamura M, Omiya Y, Higuchi M, Hagiwara N, Mitsuyoshi S, Toda H, Saito T, Tanichi M, Yoshino A, Tokuno S (2021) Depressive mood assessment method based on emotion

level derived from voice: comparison of voice features of individuals with major depressive disorders and healthy controls. Int J Environ Res Public Health 18(10):5435
United Nations Population Division (2002) World population ageing: 1950–2050. Global Action on Aging, New York

Chapter 11
Depression: Multiple Regression

Mitsuteru Nakamura

A clinical examination allows clinicians to first make a qualitative diagnosis. However, in clinical practice, the same disease is often classified into different stages according to the degree to which its symptoms threaten the patient's health, progress of the disease, or difficulty of its treatment. The severity of such diseases is quantitatively assessed with interval or ordinal scales in the form of biomarkers known to be closely related to the disease or scores given in questionnaires or check sheets. In other cases, as in the concept of "me-byo," it may be more appropriate to view healthy and sick individuals as a continuum of change rather than to divide them into groups with definite diagnostic criteria. In such cases, a model that estimates the severity of the disease rather than merely the presence or absence of the disease would be more useful as it aims to predict existing quantitative indicators rather than discriminate between two or multiple groups.

Such models are generally referred to as regression models. Numerous methods have been proposed to obtain regression models. Among them, multiple regression analysis, which is considered to be a relatively classical method, is simple to perform; however, the features used in the model are expected to have some degree of correlation with the target variable to be explained by the model. By using features that are intrinsically correlated with the target variable, a robust predictive model can be obtained even for unknown data. However, it is necessary to limit the number of explanatory variables used in the model to avoid overfitting when the sample size of the data used for training is small and the number of candidate explanatory variables is large. This issue is general, not limited to the multiple regression.

In this study, as a method for narrowing down the candidate explanatory variables, feature selection was conducted using the following procedure. The

M. Nakamura (✉)
Department of Bioengineering, Graduate School of Engineering, The University of Tokyo, Bunkyo-ku, Tokyo, Japan
e-mail: nakamura@bioeng.t.u-tokyo.ac.jp

S. Tokuno, H. Nakamura (eds.), *Voice Biomarkers*,
https://doi.org/10.1007/978-981-96-3109-4_11

following criteria 1 and 2 were used to reduce the number of features preliminary for enabling of multiple regression analysis.

1. Elimination of features that have zero variance in all samples (essentially, the elimination of features that cannot be explanatory variables. This criterion is not limited to regression analysis).
2. Exclusion of highly collinear features. A correlation matrix is created among the features, and the features in the highly collinear combinations are excluded except one feature. As long as the features are highly collinear with each other, it is not essential for the predictive ability of the model to decide which feature should be retained; however, if possible, it is desirable that the feature itself easily explain the phenomenon in a nonnumerical semantic way. In some cases, after the final model is obtained, it is considerable to replace the selected features with features that are highly collinear and more easily explain their meaning.

The following procedures 3, 4, and 5 are repeated until the criteria are met using the features selected above as candidate explanatory variables.

3. Execution of multiple regression analysis with the selected explanatory variables.
4. Calculation of the significance level of the features used in the model obtained from the multiple regression analysis.
5. Removal of the features with significance levels that do not meet the abovementioned criteria.

In this iterative process, the model is considered to have converged when no features are found to be removed from the model by the test. Figure 11.1 is a schematic of this algorithm.

Another method for reducing the number of features used in the model as much as possible is selecting a limited number of features using LASSO regression (Tibshirani 1996). LASSO regression builds models with fewer features by penalizing the number of features by the size of the regularization term. To ensure that an excessively large number of features are not used in the model, it is common to both calculate an information criterion, such as the Akaike information criterion (AIC) (Akaike 1974) and optimize the model in which this criterion is as low as possible. However, when the number of candidate features is large, the model with the smallest AIC is often an overfitting model with only one feature less than the number of samples.

We attempted to construct a model for predicting the severity of major depression using this approach. In the case of major depression, the Hamilton Depression Rating Scale (HDRS, or HAM-D) (Hamilton 1960), which is employed through a structured interview by a physician to assess the severity of depression in a patient, the General Healthcare Questionnaire (GHQ), Beck Depression Inventory (BDI) (Beck et al. 1961), and Patient Health Questionnaire (PHQ) (Kroenke et al. 2001) are used. These are systems for scoring the severity of depression and can be said to have an interval scale aspect.

The HAM-D is administered by physicians and is considered to be highly reliable, but the hurdles to its implementation are high. The GHQ, BDI and PHQ are

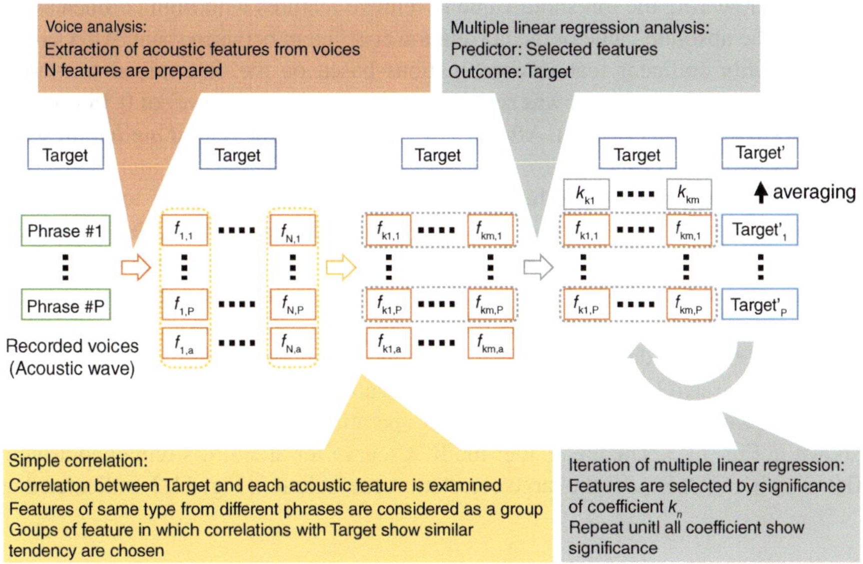

Fig. 11.1 Schematic of the algorithm for multiple regression with large number features. Annotations are as follows: *f* variable for the acoustic features, *N* number of features, *n* index of the features, *P* number of phrases, *a* index for the mean between phrases

self-administered questionnaires, and although reporting bias is a concern, there are few obstacles to their implementation. Furthermore, many examples of their use have been reported in studies. Our research group used the HAM-D to assess the severity of major depression in patients with major depression. We also used self-administered questionnaires in studies of other disorders, to identify comorbid depression and participants who are in a high-stress state prior to major depression. From these data, we constructed a prediction model wherein the features obtained from the participant's voice were used as explanatory variables and various depression scores were used as objective variables.

The study participants were recruited from outpatient clinics and had been diagnosed with major depression or bipolar disorder at National Defense Medical College Hospital (Tokorozawa, Japan). Participants were asked to read 17 specific sentences and vocalize 3 types of sustained vowels. The severity of the participants' depression was also assessed using the HAM-D. In this study, all the participants were patients with major depression or bipolar disorder and could not be distinguished from healthy controls. In contrast, the severity of depression in all the study participants, including those with bipolar disorder, was assessed using the HAM-D. After data collection, the read speech was divided by a research assistant into each sentence as a feature extraction unit. From the divided speech data, 6552 features were calculated using openSMILE (Eyben et al. 2013). The algorithm described above was applied to these features. After removing the features that did not contribute to any discrimination, we repeated multiple regression analysis by gradually lowering the threshold value to remove features with high collinearity in terms of the absolute value of the correlation coefficient between them. After eliminating highly collinear feature combinations based on the determined threshold, multiple regression analysis was repeated with a significance level of 0.1 or less as the feature selection criterion. After seven iterations, all the remaining features satisfied the selection criterion.

The relationship between the actual HAM-D score with respect to the sample used in the model construction and the HAM-D score predicted by the model obtained with this method is shown in Fig. 11.2. The correlation coefficient between the physician-rated HAM-D score and the model prediction was 0.832.

When considering the stratification of participants using cutoffs for the HAM-D (Blacker 2000), the degree of agreement between the results of stratification based on physician-rated HAM-D scores and stratification based on the index obtained by the model was evaluated using the receiver operating characteristic (ROC) curve, as shown in Fig. 11.3. The area under the ROC curve for all cutoffs remained around 0.9, which, together with the large correlation coefficient in Fig. 11.2, indicated that

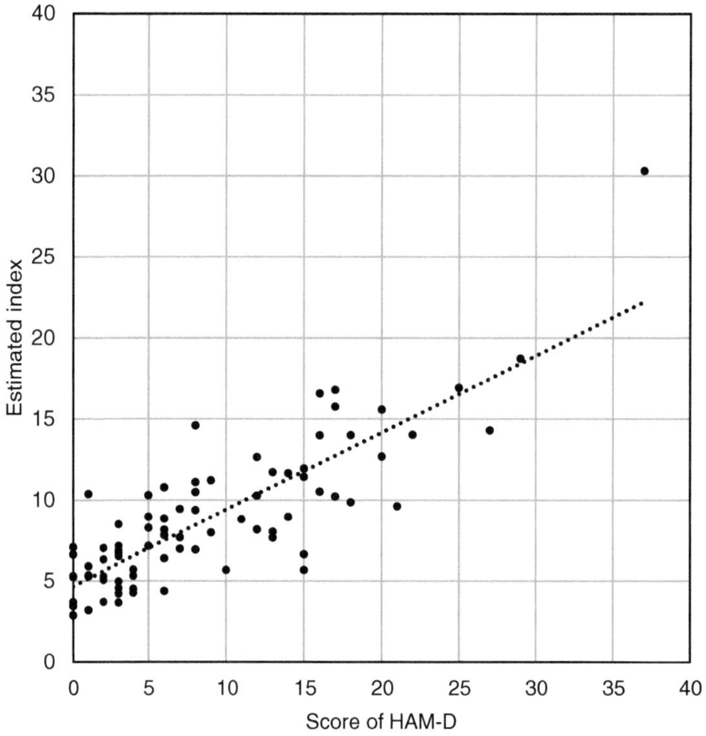

Fig. 11.2 Scatterplot between the HAM-D score evaluated by doctors and the index estimated from the patients' voices. The dotted line shows the regression line. The correlation coefficient was 0.832. (Modified from Nakamura et al. 2018)

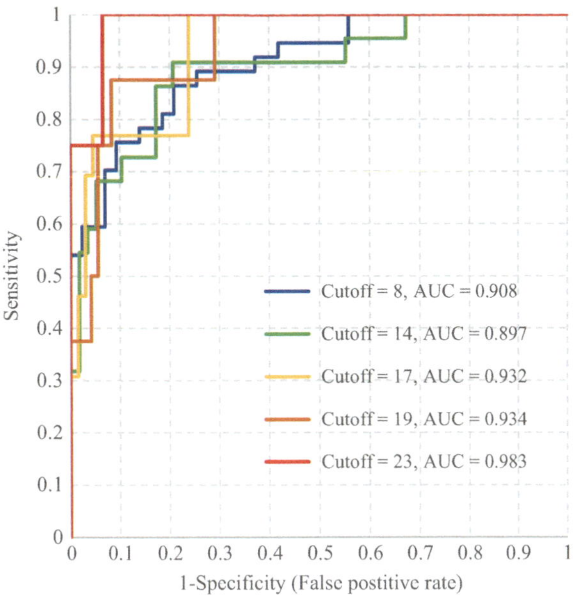

Fig. 11.3 Receiver operating characteristic curve for several cutoffs of the HAM-D score. Area under the ROC curve (AUC) for each cutoff is shown in the legend

the magnitude relationship between the physician-assessed HAM-D and the index inferred by the model was in good agreement.

We believe that these results indicate that the model obtained by multiple regression analysis of acoustic features can be used to infer not only the presence or absence of major depression but also its severity.

References

Akaike H (1974) A new look at the statistical model identification. IEEE Trans Autom Control 19(6):716–723

Beck AT, Ward CH, Mendelson M, Mock J, Erbaugh J (1961) An inventory for measuring depression. Arch Gen Psychiatry 4(6):561–571

Blacker D (2000) Psychiatric rating scales. In: Sadock B, Sadock V (eds) Comprehensive textbook of psychiatry. Lippincott Williams & Wilkins, Philadelphia, pp 755–783

Eyben F, Weninger F, Gross F, Schuller B (2013) Recent developments in openSMILE, the Munich open-source multimedia feature extractor. In: Proceedings of the 21st ACM international conference on Multimedia, Barcelona, 21–25 October 2013, pp 835–838

Hamilton M (1960) A rating scale for depression. J Neurol Neurosurg Psychiatry 23:56–62

Kroenke K, Spitzer RL, Williams JB (2001) The PHQ-9: validity of a brief depression severity measure. J Gen Intern Med 16(9):606–613

Nakamura M, Shinohara S, Omiya Y, Higuchi M, Mitsuyoshi S, Takano T, Toda H, Saito T, Tanichi M, Yoshino A, Tokuno S (2018) Feasibility study for estimation of depression severity using voice analysis, In: Proceedings of the 2018 IEEE international conference on bioinformatics and biomedicine (BIBM2018), Madrid, 3–6 December 2018

Tibshirani R (1996) Regression shrinkage and selection via the lasso. J R Stat Soc Ser B Methodol 58(1):267–288

Chapter 12
Bipolar Disorder

Masakazu Higuchi

12.1 Introduction

Depression is classified into bipolar disorder and major depressive disorder depending on the appearance of symptoms. Bipolar disorder is a psychiatric disorder with recurrent phases of mania and depression (American Psychiatric Association 2013), and distinguishing bipolar disorder from unipolar major depressive disorder during the depressive phase is difficult. Therefore, a facile method to distinguish between depression in bipolar disorder from depression in major depressive disorder is required.

12.2 Detection of Bipolar Disorder with MIMOSYS

Bipolar disorder can be classified into two types: type I with severe mania and type II with mild mania (American Psychiatric Association 2013). We first examined whether type I bipolar disorder could be detected from vitality, an indicator on the Mind Monitoring System (MIMOSYS) (Shinohara et al. 2021).

Higuchi et al. conducted a voice analysis using MIMOSYS on 25 patients (13 males, 12 females) diagnosed with type I bipolar disorder by a physician (Higuchi et al. 2019c). Voice recordings of fixed Japanese phrases were recorded in a hospital examination room using a Portable Recorder R-26 (Roland, Japan). In addition, the physician administered the Hamilton Depression Rating Scale (HDRS) (Hamilton 1960) to patients, and the patients completed a self-administered questionnaire that

M. Higuchi (✉)
Department of Bioengineering, Graduate School of Engineering, The University of Tokyo, Bunkyo-ku, Tokyo, Japan
e-mail: higuchi@bioeng.t.u-tokyo.ac.jp

S. Tokuno, H. Nakamura (eds.), *Voice Biomarkers*,
https://doi.org/10.1007/978-981-96-3109-4_12

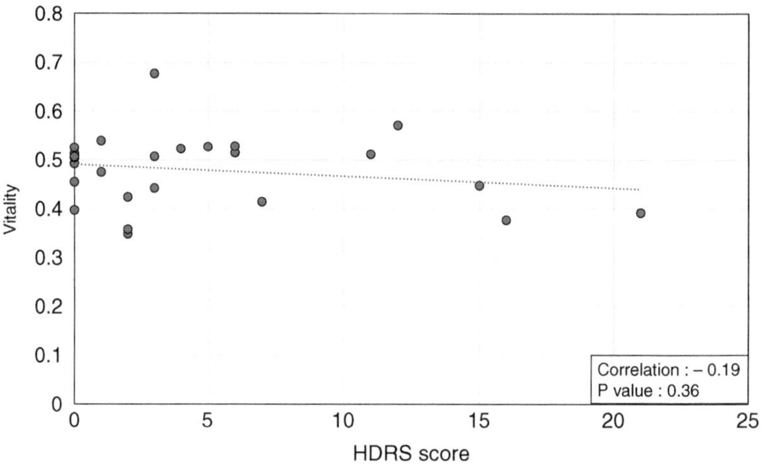

Fig. 12.1 Scatterplot of HDRS score and vitality

determined the severity of bipolar disorder based on the Young Mania Rating Scale (YMRS) (Young et al. 1978).

Figure 12.1 illustrates a scatterplot of the HDRS score and vitality, and Fig. 12.2 depicts a scatterplot of the YMRS score and vitality. No significant correlation was found between the HDRS score and vitality; however, a negative correlation ($r = -0.49$, $p = 0.012$) was found between the YMRS score and vitality. Therefore, our results suggest that vitality may be effective in detecting bipolar disorder.

12.3 Differentiation Between Bipolar Disorder and Major Depressive Disorder Using Voice Features

It is often difficult to differentiate between major depression and the depressive phase of bipolar disorder using the vitality indicator of MIMOSYS. Therefore, we attempted to follow an exploratory approach that combined multiple voice features to form a discriminant index for each disorder (Higuchi et al. 2018). First, we targeted groups consisting of healthy participants, patients with bipolar disorder, and patients with major depressive disorder. A new voice evaluation index was proposed to classify the three groups using multinomial logistic regression analysis (Agresti 2012).

The study comprised of patients visiting a hospital for treatment of bipolar disorder and major depressive disorder. Patients were diagnosed using the Mini-International Neuropsychiatric Interview: M.I.N.I. (Sheehan et al. 1998). Control subjects were healthy individuals who were living their daily lives without any issues. From the study group, 8 patients were diagnosed with bipolar disorder (BP), 14 patients were diagnosed with major depressive disorder (MD), and 32

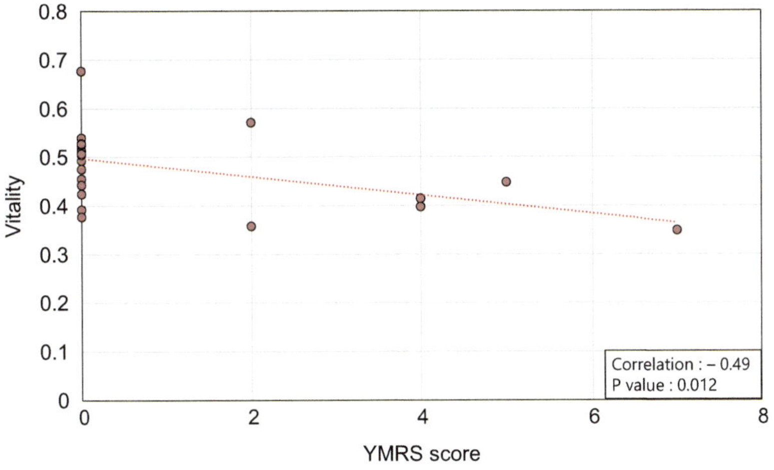

Fig. 12.2 Scatterplot of YMRS score and vitality

individuals were healthy participants (HE). In certain cases, the patients were examined multiple times, and voice recordings were recorded during each visit. We obtained 14 voice recordings from patients with bipolar disorder and 30 voice recordings from patients with major depressive disorder. Voice recordings were recorded in an examination room of the hospital, and patients were asked to read out fixed Japanese phrases. A Portable Recorder R-26 (Roland, Japan) was used for the voice recordings, and they were recorded in a 24 bit/96 kHz environment. For the extraction of features from voice, the openSMILE version 2.3 software (Eyben et al. 2010) was used. The aforementioned free software provides a set of scripts that automatically extract various feature sets from voice, and the feature set (the large openSMILE emotion feature set: emo-large) for emotion recognition was used in this study. This allowed us to extract (A) physical and similar features calculated frame-by-frame from a single voice: 56 types (fast Fourier transform, Mel-frequency cepstral coefficient, voice probability, zero crossing rate, energy, fundamental frequency, etc.), (B) temporal processing of (A): 3 types (moving average, time variation (difference), time variation of time variation), and (C) statistical quantities for each type of (B): 39 types (mean, maximum, minimum, center of gravity, quartile, variance, kurtosis, skewness, etc.), for a total of $56 \times 3 \times 39 = 6552$ voice features.

By applying multinomial logistic regression analysis using the voice features as explanatory variables, we obtained a multigroup discriminant index consisting of seven voice features. The probability of classification into three groups (P_{HE}, P_{BP}, P_{MD}) for each voice data was calculated based on the discriminant index formula, and the voice data were discriminated by classifying them into a group with the highest probability. Table 12.1 lists the discrimination results for the voice data. Overall, an accuracy of 90.79% was obtained. The discrimination probability distribution for each voice data is illustrated in Fig. 12.3. For voice data belonging to the HE group, the probability of being classified into the HE group tended to be much higher than

Table 12.1 Discrimination results of voice data

		Predicted group		
		HE	BP	MD
Actual group	HE	29	1	2
	BP	1	12	1
	MD	1	1	28

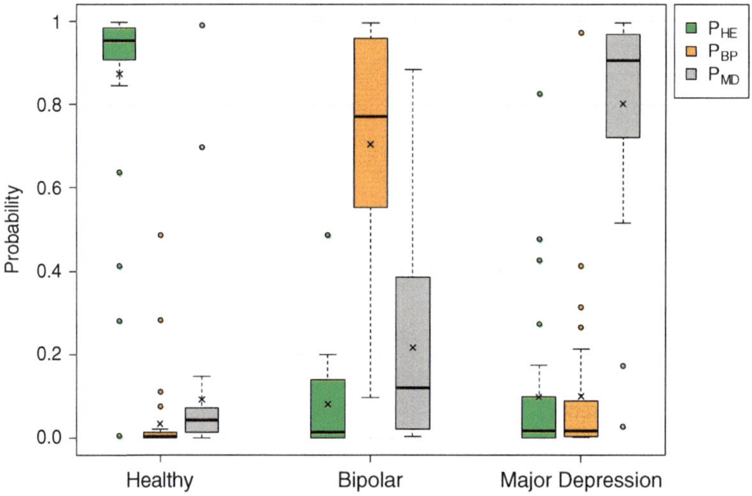

Fig. 12.3 Discriminant probability distribution of voice data. (Modified from Higuchi et al. 2018)

the probability of being classified into the other two groups. Similarly, for voice data belonging to the BP group, the probability of being classified into the BP group tended to be higher than the probability of being classified into the other two groups, although a wide range of values were noted. The probability of being classified into the MD group for voice data belonging to the MD group tended to be much higher than the probability of being classified into the other two groups. Therefore, the obtained discriminant index may serve as a new index for distinguishing bipolar disorder from major depressive disorder.

12.4 Determining the Severity of Bipolar Disorder

We propose an index to discriminate between type I and type II bipolar disorders using an exploratory approach that combines multiple voice features (Higuchi et al. 2019a, b).

This study included patients who visited a hospital for treatment of bipolar disorder. Patients were diagnosed using the M.I.N.I. Control subjects were healthy individuals who were living their daily lives without any issues. The study group comprised of 25 patients diagnosed with bipolar I disorder (BPI), 39 patients diagnosed with bipolar II disorder (BPII), and 14 healthy participants (HE). Voice recordings were recorded in a hospital examination room, and the patients were asked to read aloud fixed Japanese phrases. A Portable Recorder R-26 (Roland, Japan) was used for voice recording, and the recordings were recorded in a 24 bit/96 kHz environment. The voice data were segmented into utterance units, and feature extraction was carried out using the openSMILE version 2.3 software. From each utterance, 6552 voice features were extracted using the emo-large feature set.

For the training data, 75% of the participants were selected from the HE, BPI, and BPII groups. Regularized multinomial logistic regression analysis (Friedman et al. 2010) was performed on the voice features obtained from the voice recordings of participants as explanatory variables. This resulted in a multigroup discriminant index consisting of 196 voice features. The probability of each voice data being classified into the aforementioned three groups was calculated based on the discriminant index formula. The voice data were discriminated by classifying them into a group with the highest probability, and the group prediction for each participant was performed by voting based on the results of each voice data. For each participant, the group to which their voice data belonged was predicted based on the discriminant index, and the group with the highest number of predictions was determined as the group to which the participant belonged. If the most frequently predicted group was more than one, the participant was judged to be unknown. Table 12.2 presents the confusion matrix obtained from the group predictions for participants in the training data. Overall, a correct response rate of 96.7% was achieved. The discrimination probability distribution for each participant is presented in Fig. 12.4. This probability was calculated by dividing the voting score for each group obtained from the prediction of the participant's utterance data by the number of utterances for that particular participant. The figure indicates that for a participant belonging to the target group, the probability of being discriminated into the target group tended to be higher than the probabilities of being discriminated into the other two groups.

Table 12.3 presents the confusion matrix obtained from the group predictions for 25% of the participants (validation data), who were not included in the training data. Overall, a correct response rate of 66.7% was achieved. The discriminant probability distribution for each participant is illustrated in Fig. 12.5. The figure reveals that for a participant belonging to the HE group, the probability of being classified into the HE group tended to be higher than the probabilities of being classified into the

Table 12.2 Confusion matrix for training data participants

		Predicted group				
		HE	BPI	BPII	Unknown	Recall
Actual group	HE	10	0	1	0	90.9%
	BPI	0	18	1	0	94.7%
	BPII	0	0	30	0	100%
	Precision	100%	100%	93.8%	0%	Accuracy 96.7%

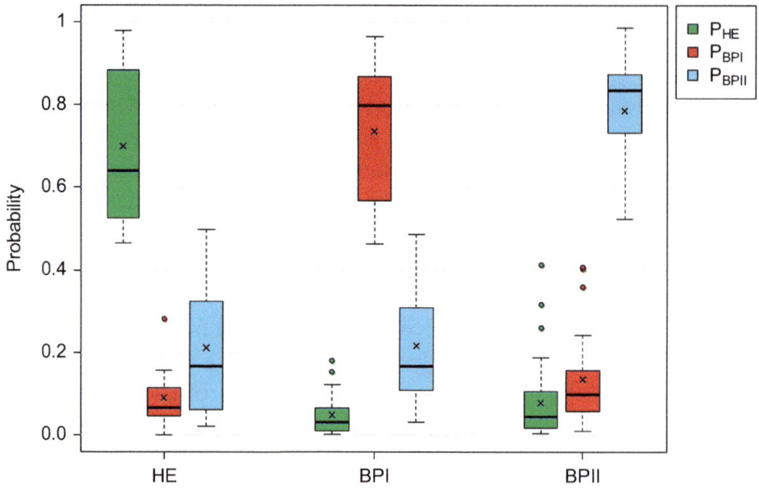

Fig. 12.4 Discriminant probability distribution of training data participants. (Modified from Higuchi et al. 2019a, b)

Table 12.3 Confusion matrix for validation data participants

		Predicted group				
		HE	BPI	BPII	Unknown	Recall
Actual group	HE	3	0	0	0	100%
	BPI	1	3	2	0	50.0%
	BPII	0	3	6	0	66.7%
	Precision	75.0%	50.0%	75.0%	0%	Accuracy 66.7%

other two groups. For participants belonging to the BPI and BPII groups, the probability of being classified into the BPI and BPII groups tended to be similar. Although the correct rate for the validation data was poor, the correct rate for the training data was significantly high, suggesting that it is possible to discriminate the severity of bipolar disorder based on speech.

12.5 Conclusion

We investigated the possibility of detection of bipolar disorder and classification of its severity based on voice data. The results suggested that the MIMOSYS technology may be effective in detecting bipolar disorder type I. However, several participants presented a YMRS score of zero, leaving room for re-examination. In an exploratory approach that combined multiple voice features, we obtained a discriminative index that accurately classified healthy, bipolar, and major depressive disorder groups. Further studies are, however, required to validate these results using

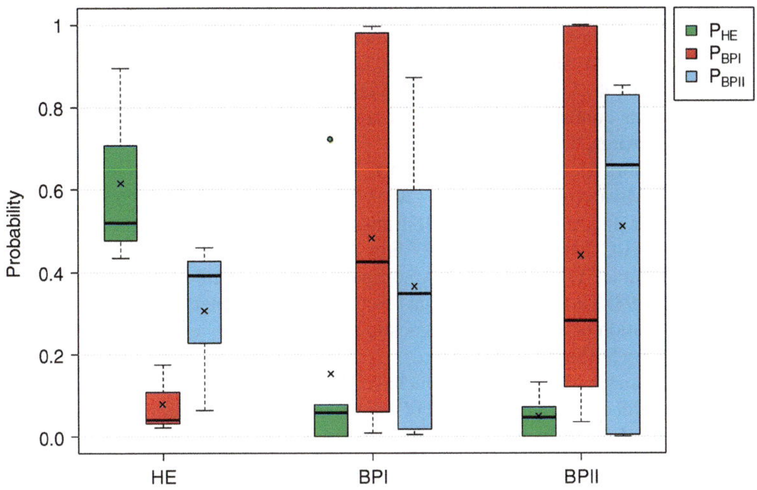

Fig. 12.5 Discriminant probability distribution of validation data participants. (Modified from Higuchi et al. 2019a, b)

other data groups. Using the same exploratory approach, we obtained an index discriminating healthy, type I, and type II bipolar disorder groups; however, its validation accuracy was low. The reason for this may be the insufficient number of data points in the validation group. Nevertheless, the correct rate in the training group was significantly high, suggesting that the possibility of classifying the severity of bipolar disorder is satisfactory.

From the above, it can be concluded that based on voice data, detecting bipolar disorder and classifying its severity to a certain extent is possible.

References

Agresti A (2012) Categorical data analysis, 3rd edn. Wiley-Interscience, New Jersey

American Psychiatric Association (2013) Diagnostic and statistical manual of mental disorders V. American Psychiatric Publications Inc, New York

Eyben F, Wöllmer M, Schuller B (2010) openSMILE—The Munich Versatile and fast open-source audio feature extractor. In: Proceedings of the 18th ACM international conference on multimedia, Firenze, 25–29 October 2010, pp 1459–1462

Friedman J, Hastie T, Tibshirani R (2010) Regularization paths for generalized linear models via coordinate descent. J Stat Softw 33(1):1–22

Hamilton M (1960) A rating scale for depression. J Neurol Neurosurg Psychiatry 23:56–62

Higuchi M, Tokuno S, Nakamura M, Shinohara S, Mitsuyoshi S, Omiya Y, Hagiwara N, Takano T, Toda H, Saito T, Terashi H, Mitoma H (2018) Classification of bipolar disorder, major depressive disorder and healthy state using voice. Asian J Pharm Clin Res 11(3):89–93

Higuchi M, Nakamura M, Shinohara S, Omiya Y, Takano T, Toda H, Saito T, Yoshino A, Mitsuyoshi S, Tokuno S (2019a) Discrimination of bipolar disorders using voice. pervasive computing paradigms for mental health. MindCare 2019. Lecture Notes of the Institute for Computer Sciences, Social Informatics and Telecommunications Engineering 288. Springer, pp 199–207

Higuchi M, Nakamura M, Shinohara S, Omiya Y, Takano T, Toda H, Saito T, Yoshino A, Mitsuyoshi S, Tokuno S (2019b) Discrimination of bipolar disorders using voice. In: Proceedings of 9th EAI international conference on pervasive computing paradigms for mental health (MindCare 2019), Buenos Aires, 23–24 April 2019

Higuchi M, Nakamura M, Shinohara S, Omiya Y, Takano T, Suzuki K, Manome N, Toda H, Saito T, Yoshino A, Mitsuyoshi S, Tokuno S (2019c) Effectiveness of voice biomarker in detecting bipolar disorder. In: Abstracts of the 41st international engineering in medicine and biology conference (EMBC 2019), Berlin, 23–27 July 2019

Sheehan DV, Lecrubier Y, Sheehan KH, Amorim P, Janavs J, Weiller E, Her-gueta T, Baker R, Dunbar GC (1998) The Mini-International Neuropsychiatric Interview (M.I.N.I): the development and validation of a structured diagnostic psychiatric interview for DSM-IV and ICD-10. J Clin Psychiatry 59(Suppl 20):22–33

Shinohara S, Nakamura M, Omiya Y, Higuchi M, Hagiwara N, Mitsuyoshi S, Toda H, Saito T, Tanichi M, Yoshino A, Tokuno S (2021) Depressive mood assessment method based on emotion level derived from voice: comparison of voice features of individuals with major depressive disorders and healthy controls. Int J Environ Res Public Health 18(10):5435

Young RC, Biggs JT, Ziegler VE, Meyer DA (1978) A rating scale for mania: reliability, validity and sensitivity. Br J Psychiatry 133(5):429–435

Chapter 13
Post-traumatic Stress Disorder (PTSD)

Masakazu Higuchi

13.1 Introduction

Body identification is a vital task after a disaster wherein dentists compare the dental findings of dead bodies with antemortem dental records and X-rays to determine the identity of the deceased individuals. Body identification is extremely stressful in disaster medicine settings and can occasionally cause severe health issues, such as post-traumatic stress disorder (PTSD) (Katayama et al. 2012; Shigemura et al. 2018; Ursano and McCarroll 1990). Although dentists receive abundant requests for assistance in postmortem examinations and autopsies, they rarely come in contact with actual dead bodies during their routine medical care duties. Therefore, they are expected to experience stress associated with body identification (McCarroll et al. 1996). Many dentists employed for body identification work after the 2011 Tohoku earthquake faced mental health issues (Shigemura et al. 2018).

To prepare for large-scale body identification during major disasters, dentists regularly undergo training using manikins or actual dead bodies at dental body identification workshops (Yamamoto et al. 2016). However, even during training, these medical professionals may experience stress due to their exposure to dead bodies. Despite this growing concern, stress levels of dentists have never been measured during body identification training. Therefore, a simple and time efficient stress assessment method is required that can be applied during the brief time available in these workshops.

In our previous study, we verified the effectiveness of stress measurement in dental body identification workshops using the mind monitoring system (MIMOSYS) (Shinohara et al. 2021).

M. Higuchi (✉)
Department of Bioengineering, Graduate School of Engineering, The University of Tokyo, Bunkyo-ku, Tokyo, Japan
e-mail: higuchi@bioeng.t.u-tokyo.ac.jp

S. Tokuno, H. Nakamura (eds.), *Voice Biomarkers*,
https://doi.org/10.1007/978-981-96-3109-4_13

13.2 Assessment of Stress Load Through Workshops

We used MIMOSYS (Omiya et al. 2017) to measure the degree of stress applied throughout the body identification workshop where actual bodies and manikins were employed during practical training sessions. Twenty-three participants, including police dentists and private dentists, attended the workshop. We recorded their voice at the beginning and end of the workshop using a portable voice recorder R-26 (Roland, Japan); the recordings were readings of fixed Japanese phrases. Furthermore, participants were asked to indicate their subjective fatigue level on a visual analog scale (VAS).

MIMOSYS is based on Sensibility Technology (ST) (Mitsuyoshi et al. 2006), which is a voice emotion recognition technology. ST analyzes change patterns in the fundamental frequency of a voice recording and detects emotional components contained in the voice, namely, "calmness," "anger," "joy," "sorrow," and "excitement." For this experiment, these emotional components were calculated using ST as well as the vitality of MIMOSYS, and the amount of change from the beginning to the end of the workshop was examined. The details are presented in Table 13.1. A significant difference ($p = 0.050$) was confirmed with the corresponding t-test for the excitement component. The excitement component tended to increase, indicating that the participants were aroused by strong mental stimulation received during the workshop. In addition to the vitality and emotional components, changes in pitch rate of voice were examined as well, and a significant difference ($p = 0.034$) was found. However, the relationship between pitch rate and stress is not clear, and the reason for the obtained difference is unknown. A positive correlation was found between change in the anger component and change in subjective fatigue from the beginning to the end of the workshop. This indicates that participants who were

Table 13.1 Measurements of emotional components, vitality, and pitch rate at the beginning and end of the workshop and their relationship to subjective fatigue level ($*p < 0.05$)

	Before workshop	After workshop		Paired t-test		Correlation between feature and VAS in difference
Features	Mean ± SD	Mean ± SD	Difference	t	*P* value	
Calmness	0.57 ± 0.11	0.57 ± 0.083	–0.0010	0.035	N.S. (0.97)	–0.060
Anger	0.088 ± 0.038	0.10 ± 0.040	0.012	–1.19	N.S. (0.25)	0.45
Joy	0.17 ± 0.16	0.18 ± 0.083	0.0010	–0.037	N.S. (0.97)	–0.020
Sorrow	0.17 ± 0.084	0.15 ± 0.078	–0.013	0.63	N.S. (0.53)	–0.11
Excitement	0.20 ± 0.22	0.082 ± 0.095	0.023	–2.07	0.050*	–0.080
Vitality	0.50 ± 0.56	0.24 ± 0.19	0.056	–0.93	N.S. (0.36)	–0.030
Pitch rate	0.51 ± 0.56	0.15 ± 0.15	0.050	–2.27	0.034*	–0.090

angry at the end of the workshop felt more fatigued and may have been irritated or tired during the workshop for reasons unknown. These results suggest the possibility of using voice to estimate degree of fatigue in participants.

13.3 Assessment of Stress Load During Training Using Dead Bodies

Since exposure to stress was expected in the body identification workshop, in particular during practical training sessions using actual dead bodies, we examined the mental status of the participants before and after training using dead bodies (Higuchi et al. 2017a, b; Yamamoto et al. 2018). This training workshop contained 27 participants, namely, police dentists and private dentists, and included practical training using actual bodies and manikins. The participants were divided into several groups, and training was conducted such that there was no overlap in the training content between the groups. We focused on a group that used an actual dead body in the first training after the workshop began (A: 10 participants) and a group that trained with a manikin prior to training with an actual dead body (B: 17 participants). We recorded the voices of the participants of each group before and after they underwent training with the dead body. The recordings were readings of fixed Japanese phrases and were recorded using a portable recorder R-26 (Roland, Japan).

Figure 13.1 displays the results of the change in vitality for groups A and B; the vertical axis indicates the rate of change of vitality based on before training with the dead body. In group A, MIMOSYS analysis revealed a remarkable difference in change in vitality before and after training with dead bodies; in contrast, in group B, the change in vitality was nearly identical. The change in vitality for group A was in the direction of increase. A report has stated that subjects get temporarily excited immediately after being exposed to strong stress (Herman and Cullinan 1977); therefore, the increase in vitality in group A after training with dead bodies was considered to be representative of elevated mood due to stress. In group B, manikin training may have improved stress tolerance toward the first exposure of the

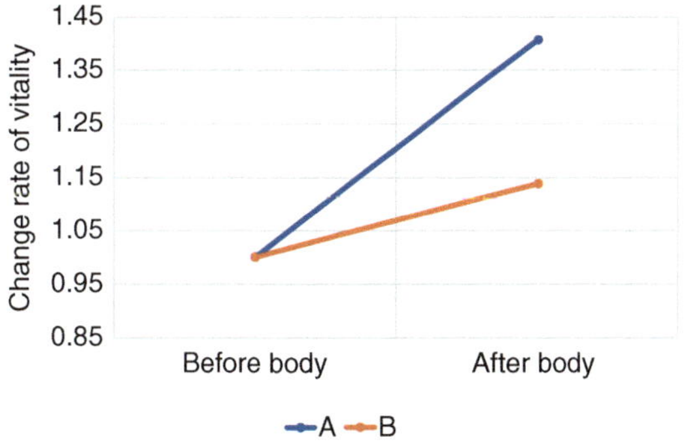

Fig. 13.1 Rate of change in vitality before and after training with dead bodies

participants to dead bodies, confirming the effectiveness of the workshop with respect to stress exposure.

13.4 Assessment of Stress Load With and Without On-Site Experience

In the experiment discussed in Sect. 13.3, due to a biased distribution of participants with and without on-site body identification experience, we were unable to identify whether the change in the mental state of the two groups was due to the manikin experience or the presence or absence of actual previous experience. Regarding previous experience, a report has stated that emergency personnel who did not undergo specialist training developed PTSD at higher rates than those who underwent training (Hagh-Shenas et al. 2005), thereby suggesting that previous experience or lack thereof has an impact on stress levels. Therefore, we investigated the effects of having/not having actual experience and undergoing/not undergoing previous training (that is, training prior to dead body training) on the mental state of participants during the workshop (Higuchi et al. 2019, 2020).

This workshop involved practical training using actual bodies, manikins, and case files. Training with case files involved formulating findings based on photographs of actual bodies. The participants were divided into three groups (A, B, and C), and the groups were rotated to avoid duplicate training. Table 13.2 shows the training order of the groups during the workshop. As per the table, the order of practical training for group A was dead body, case file, and manikin; group B was manikin, dead body, and case file; and group C was case file, manikin, and dead body. The voices of the participants were recorded before and after each training session wherein they read a fixed phrase in Japanese. The workshop consisted of 129 participants, including police dentists (44), independent dentists (8), Japan Dental Association members (32), police staff (21), Japan Coast Guard staff (2), Japan Self-Defense Force members (4), university staff (16), and others (6). Four respondents belonged to multiple organizations. Group A, B, and C consisted of 45, 40, and 44 subjects, respectively. Participants who confirmed actual experience in body identification were yes: 17, no: 25 in group A; yes: 12, no: 20 in group B; and yes: 16, no: 24 in group C. We studied whether two factors, namely actual previous experience of body identification and type of prior training, had an impact on the mental state when they were independent or when they interacted with each other, that is, there was some overlap of the two factors. To this end, we performed a

Table 13.2 Training order for each group

Group	First training	Second training	Third training
A	Body	Case file	Manikin
B	Manikin	Body	Case file
C	Case file	Manikin	Body

two-way analysis of variance (ANOVA) on the absolute difference in vitality before and after training using a dead body.

The mean absolute differences in vitality for each group are displayed in Fig. 13.2. Prior to dead body training, group A underwent none, group B underwent manikin training, and group C underwent case file and manikin training. The solid line exp(+) represents the line connecting the mean of the absolute difference in vitality of subjects with actual experience for each group, and the dotted line exp(−) represents the line connecting the mean of the absolute difference in vitality of subjects without actual experience for each group. ANOVA results, considering the factors of presence or absence of actual experience in body identification and type of prior training, did not provide a significant effect for either experience or prior training. In other words, regardless of the type of prior training, there was no difference in the absolute difference in vitality between those with and without experience. Similarly, regardless of experience, there was no difference in the absolute difference in vitality between types of prior training. However, a significant interaction ($p = 0.030$) between the two factors was confirmed, suggesting that the presence or absence of actual experience and the type of prior training interacted to influence a change in mental state before and after dead body training. Focusing on the type of prior training, the absolute difference in vitality between pre- and post-training was smaller for participants in exp(−) of group B than those for exp(+) of group B. Furthermore, a significant difference ($p = 0.022$) between the two absolute differences in vitality was confirmed. Focusing on experience, for the exp(-) group, a significant difference ($p = 0.0079$) was confirmed between the types of prior

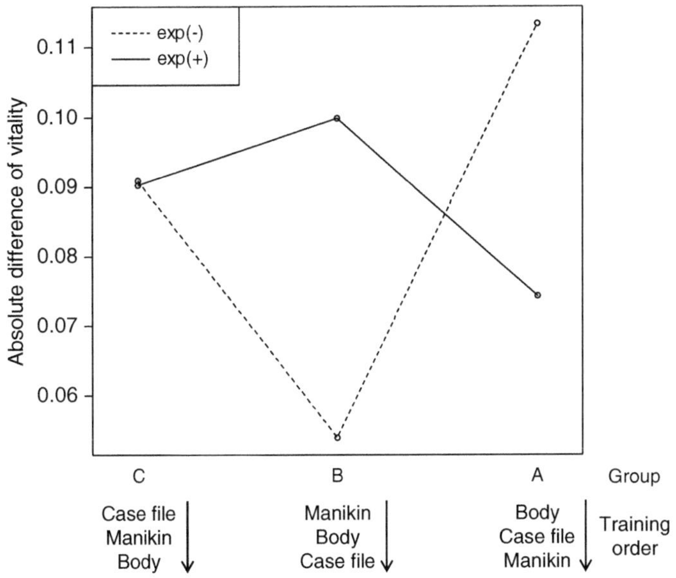

Fig. 13.2 Mean absolute differences in vitality between pre- and post-training for each group. (Modified from Higuchi et al. 2020)

training, in particular between group A without prior training and group B with prior training involving manikins ($p = 0.0057$). The absolute difference in vitality was much smaller for group B with prior training using manikins than that for group A without any prior training. These results suggest that prior manikin training increases stress resilience for participants coming into contact with dead bodies for the first time, confirming the effectiveness of the workshop in stress exposure. For exp(−), similar results were obtained for group C with prior training using case files and manikins; however, the absolute difference in vitality was smaller for this group than that for group A without any prior training, and the difference was not significant. The absolute difference in vitality for group C with prior training using case files and manikins was larger than that for group B with prior training using manikins. We believe that this is due to the impact of training with case files and suggest the possibility that just seeing photographs of dead bodies leads to stress exposure. In other words, stress levels are highest during involvement with dead bodies, followed by photographs and manikins. The abovementioned results demonstrate that changes occur in the mental state pre- and post-training depending on the presence or absence of actual body identification experience and type of prior training.

13.5 Conclusion

We investigated the differences in the stress levels of participants in dental body identification workshops, which are held regularly for dentists and related personnel, using voice stress measurement, depending on their actual experience and the training order. The results of the evaluation of changes in mental state before and after dead body training using the vitality of MIMOSYS suggested that mental state changed depending on the experience of body identification in the actual setting and the type of prior training before the dead body training. Furthermore, the results suggest that prior manikin training may improve stress tolerance for participants when they come in contact with a dead body for the first time. The effectiveness of manikin training for stress exposure was confirmed as well. Moreover, the voice stress assessment technique was easy to use and could be conducted in a limited time during the training. Furthermore, it could verify a certain effect of the workshop. Therefore, it can be useful in an actual disaster site.

References

Hagh-Shenas H, Goodarzi MA, Dehbozorgi G, Farashbandi H (2005) Psychological consequences of the Bam earthquake on professional and nonprofessional helpers. J Trauma Stress 18(5):477–483

Herman JP, Cullinan WE (1977) Neurocircuitry of stress: central control of the hypothalamo–pituitary–adrenocortical axis. Trends Neurosci 20(2):78–84

Higuchi M, Yamamoto I, Shinohara S, Nakamura M, Omiya Y, Hagiwara H, Takano T, Mitsuyoshi S, Tokuno S (2017a) Stress level measurement using voice for mental care in body identification work [Translated from Japanese]. In: Abstract of Japanese Bio-Medical Engineering Symposium (JBMES 2017), Ueda, 15–16 September 2017 (in Japanese)

Higuchi M, Yamamoto I, Omiya Y, Shinohara S, Nakamura M, Hagiwara N, Takano T, Mitsuyoshi S, Tokuno S (2017b) Measurement of stress level to prevent post-traumatic stress disorder developed by identifying dead bodies. Econophys Sociophys Other Multidiscip Sci J 7(1):13–18

Higuchi M, Yamamoto I, Omiya Y, Nakamura M, Shinohara S, Takano T, Nakagawa K, Ohira H, Yamada Y, Hasegawa I, Mitsuyoshi S, Tokuno S (2019) Voice-based evaluation of stress by body identification. In: Abstract of 26th international "stress and behavior" neuroscience and biopsychiatry conference (ISBS 2019), St. Petersburg, 16–19 May 2019

Higuchi M, Yamamoto I, Omiya Y, Nakamura M, Shinohara S, Takano T, Nakagawa K, Ohira H, Yamada Y, Tokuno S (2020) Effects of long- and short-term experiences on stress during identification works of dead bodies: rapid stress level measurement using voice. Am J Disaster Med 15(4):251–259

Katayama K, Itoga H, Someda H (2012) Lessons learned from dental activities in the Great East Japan Earthquake disaster relief mission (First Report): disaster victim identification activities conducted by Japan Self-Defense Forces Dental Officers [Translated from Japanese]. Nat Defense Med J 59(12):131–139. (in Japanese)

McCarroll JE, Fullerton CS, Ursano RJ, Hermsen JM (1996) Posttraumatic stress symptoms following forensic dental identification: Mt. Carmel, Waco, Texas. Am J Psychiatry 153(6):778–782

Mitsuyoshi S, Ren F, Tanaka Y, Kuroiwa S (2006) Non-verbal voice emotion analysis system. Int J Innov Comput Inf Control 2(4):819–830

Omiya Y, Shinohara S, Higuchi M, Nakamura M, Mitsuyoshi S, Yamamoto I, Tokuno S (2017) Stress evaluation using voice in dental identification work of dead body. In: Abstract of neuroscience 2017, Washington, 11–15 November 2017

Shigemura J, Someda H, Tokuno S, Nagamine M, Tanichi M, Araki Y, Nagakawa S, Saito T, Tsumatori G, Itabashi J, Kanno A (2018) Disaster victim identification: psychological distress and posttraumatic stress in dentists after the 2011 Fukushima disaster. Psychiatry 81(1):85–92

Shinohara S, Nakamura M, Omiya Y, Higuchi M, Hagiwara N, Mitsuyoshi S, Toda H, Saito T, Tanichi M, Yoshino A, Tokuno S (2021) Depressive mood assessment method based on emotion level derived from voice: comparison of voice features of individuals with major depressive disorders and healthy controls. Int J Environ Res Public Health 18(10):5435

Ursano RJ, McCarroll JE (1990) The nature of a traumatic stressor: handling dead bodies. J Nerv Ment Dis 178(6):396–398

Yamamoto I, Ohira H, Yamada Y, Kimoto K, Nihei T, Hamada N, Lee M, Tsukinoki K (2016) Identification training program using a cadaver-like dental mannequin [Translated from Japanese]. Jpn J Disaster Med 21(2):173–178. (in Japanese)

Yamamoto I, Higuchi M, Tokuno S, Ohira H, Yamado Y, Kimoto K, Nihei T, Hamada N, Lee M, Tsukinoki K (2018) A study of stress measurement for mental health care in dental identification training [Translated from Japanese]. In: Abstract of the 23nd annual meeting of Japanese Association for Disaster Medicine, Yokohama, 1 February 2018 (in Japanese)

Chapter 14
Parkinson's Disease

Shuji Shinohara

14.1 Introduction

With the aging of society, the prevalence of dementia and Parkinson's disease is increasing. Early detection and preventive treatment of these diseases are important to address this problem. Most Parkinson's patients have some form of movement disorder, and regular visits to the hospital can be burdensome for the patient and their family. It is also estimated that 90% of patients with Parkinson's disease have some type of speech disorder. Our research aimed to use voice to estimate health status. Voice analysis has the advantage of being noninvasive and can be remotely controlled using a smartphone or other devices. If Parkinson's disease patients' conditions can be monitored remotely, it will reduce the burden of patient visits to the hospital.

In this chapter, we present two speech metrics that can discriminate between normal subjects and patients with Parkinson's disease (PWPD) and one speech metric that can identify the severity of Parkinson's disease. One index discriminates between normal and PWPD using two features: Hurst exponent (HE) and zero crossing rate (ZCR) (Parkinson's Disease Voice Index (PDVI)). The openSMILE features were utilized for the other discriminant index between healthy subjects and PWPD and a severity index.

S. Shinohara (✉)
Division of Information Systems and Design, School of Science and Engineering, Tokyo Denki University, Hiki-gun, Saitama, Japan
e-mail: s.shinohara@mail.dendai.ac.jp

S. Tokuno, H. Nakamura (eds.), *Voice Biomarkers*,
https://doi.org/10.1007/978-981-96-3109-4_14

14.2 Speech Data of Patients with Parkinson's Disease and Normal Subjects

We collected 14 Japanese standardized speech utterances and 3 types of long vowels (Ah, Eh, Uh) from PWPD attending a university hospital and healthy subjects to create the speech indexes described above. Speech utterances of PWPD and healthy subjects were recorded in the same examination room. Table 14.1 shows the contents of the standardized phrases. Table 14.2 presents the subject information.

A portable recorder R-26 (Roland, Japan) was used for voice recording. The sampling frequency was 96 KHz and the quantization bit rate was 24 bits. Voice was manually segmented into speech units.

The severity of PWPD was scored by a physician at the time of voice recording using a modified version of the Hoehn and Yahr stage. One patient had stage 1 disease (henceforth, PD1), 13 patients had stage 2 disease (henceforth, PD2), 3 patients had stage 2.5 (henceforth, PD2.5), and 3 patients had stage 3 disease (henceforth, PD3).

14.3 Parkinson's Disease Voice Index (PDVI) Using Hurst Index and Zero Crossing Rate

PDVI uses two features: the Hurst exponent (HE) and zero crossing rate (ZCR). Refer to Chap. 7 for details on the calculation of HE and ZCR from the speech waveforms.

Table 14.1 Fourteen canned phrases used in the analysis

Phrase	Phrase in Japanese	Purpose (meaning)
P1	I-ro-ha-ni-ho-he-to	Nonemotional (no meaning, similar to "a-b-c")
P2	Honjitsu ha seiten nari	Nonemotional (It is fine today)
P3	Tsurezurenarumamani	Nonemotional (at a loose end)
P4	Wagahaiha neko dearu	Nonemotional (I am a cat)
P5	Mukashi aru tokoro ni	Nonemotional (Once upon a time, there lived)
P6	Aiueo Gagigugego Rarirurero Papipupepo	Check pronunciation
P7	Omoeba tokue kitamonda	Nonemotional (We've come a long way, come to think of it)
P8	Garapagosu shotou	Check pronunciation (Galápagos Islands)
P9	Tsukarete guttari shiteimasu.	Emotional (I am tired/dead tired)
P6	Totemo genki desu	Emotional (I am very cheerful)
P11	Kinou ha yoku nemuremashita	Emotional (I was able to sleep well yesterday)
P12	Shokuyoku ga arimasu	Emotional (I have an appetite)
P13	Okorippoi desu	Emotional (I am irritable)
P14	Kokoroga odayaka desu	Emotional (My heart is calm)

Table 14.2 Subject information

Subject type	Sex	Number of subjects
PWPD	Female	8
	Male	12
	Total	20
Healthy	Female	13
	Male	19
	Total	32

HE is a widely used index in the field of stock price analysis for measuring the long-term memory characteristics of a time series (Eom et al. 2008). HE considers values in the range (0.0, 1.0) and is small for complex waveforms, such as white noise, and close to 1.0 for smooth waveforms, such as sine waves. Let D be the fractal dimension of the signal waveform and HE be represented by HE = 2 − D. In other words, HE can be regarded as an index of waveform smoothness (the inverse of fractal dimension).

ZCR, on the other hand, is an index commonly used in studies on voice activity detection and voiced/unvoiced sound classification, which indicates the rate at which the signal changes from positive to negative or vice versa (Jalil et al. 2013; Bachu et al. 2010; Kazi et al. 2017). In contrast to HE, ZCR tends to be larger for complex waveforms and smaller for smooth waveforms. We focused on the relationship between HE and ZCR as a speech index that can discriminate between healthy subjects and PWPD.

Figure 14.1 shows the scatterplots of HE and ZCR calculated from healthy and PWPD speeches. It can be observed that both fixed phrases and long vowels tend to be distributed in the upper right of the straight line ZCR = 0.23HE + 0.215 for patient speech and in the lower left for normal speech. Based on this trend, we defined PDVI as follows:

Figure 14.2 shows a comparison of the PDVI between healthy subjects and PWPD. In the case of the fixed phrases, the PDVI means ± SD of healthy subjects and PWPD were −0.011 ± 0.0084 ($n = 32$) and 0.014 ± 0.012 ($n = 15$), respectively. A t-test showed a significant difference between the two groups at the 1% level of significance.

In the case of long vowels, the PDVI means ± SD of healthy subjects and PWPD were −0.010 ± 0.0077 ($n = 32$) and 0.0044 ± 0.012 ($n = 15$), respectively. The t-test results showed a significant difference between the two groups at the 1% level.

The AUC for PDVI discrimination between normal subjects and PWPD in the fixed phrases was 0.975, and sensitivity and specificity were 0.906 and 1.000, respectively. In contrast, for long vowels, the AUC, sensitivity, and specificity were 0.883, 0.906, and 0.800, respectively, when PDVI discriminated between normal subjects and PWPD. A summary of the results is presented in Table 14.3.

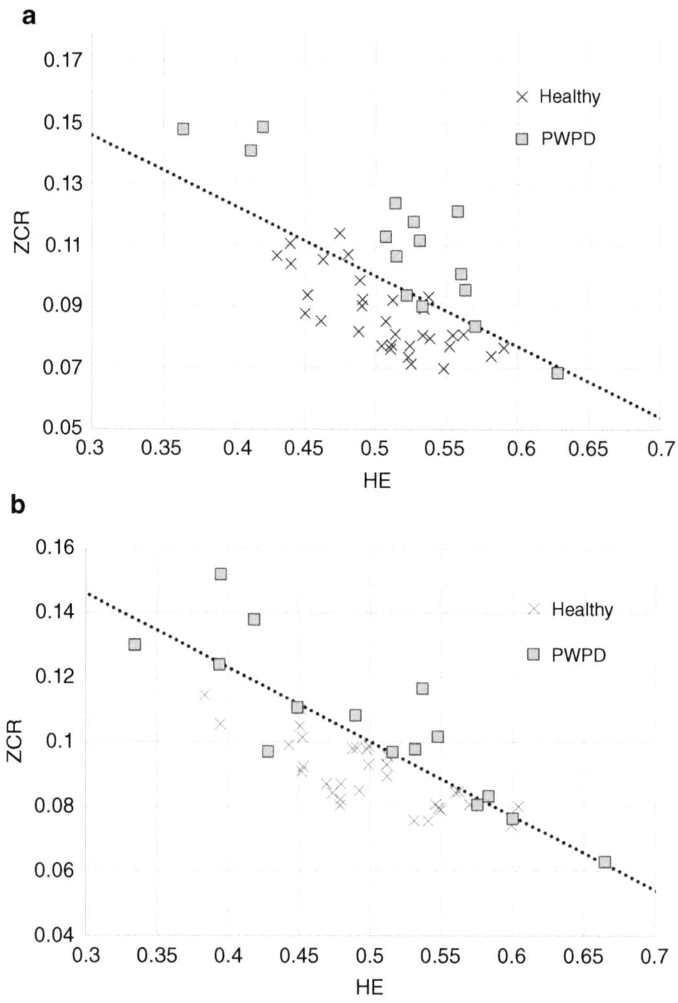

Fig. 14.1 Scatterplot of Hurst index and zero crossing rate calculated from normal and PWPD speech. The figure also shows the straight line ZCR = 0.23HE + 0.215. (**a**) Fixed phrases. (**b**) Long vowels

14.4 Speech Index for Parkinson's Disease Identification Using openSMILE

In this section, we present a speech index for discriminating healthy subjects from PWPD and a speech index for identifying the severity of Parkinson's disease using the free software openSMILE (Eyben et al. 2010).

Only regular phrase utterances of the patients' speech were used for speech. For both indices, openSMILE version 2.3 was used to extract speech features, and 6552

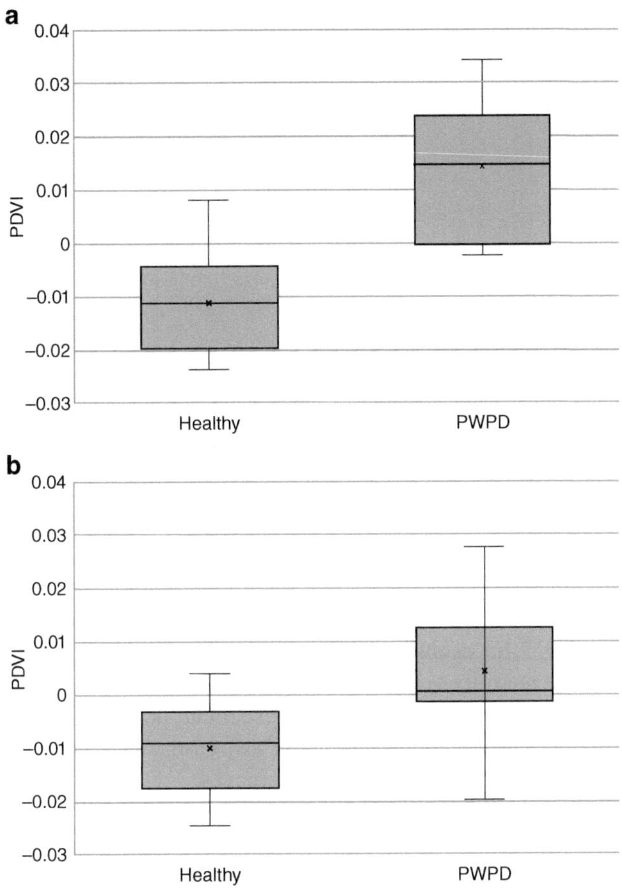

Fig. 14.2 Boxplots of PDVI computed from normal and PWPD speech. (**a**) Fixed phrases. (**b**) Long vowels

Table 14.3 Discrimination performance of PDVI between healthy subjects and patients

Speech type	AUC	Sensitivity	Specificity
Fixed phrase	0.975	0.906	1.000
Long vowel	0.883	0.906	0.800

speech features were extracted from a single utterance using the feature set used in emotion recognition (the large openSMILE emotion feature set).

The bagging (J48) classification algorithm (implemented in Weka) was developed to classify healthy participants and PWPD by using approximately three-quarters of the subject's speech.

For healthy participants and PWPD, validation was performed using the remaining one-quarter of the subject's speech not used in the algorithm creation. The

Table 14.4 Discrimination results for speech data

		Predict				Recall
		PD1	PD2	PD2.5	PD3	
Actual	PD1	30	6	0	0	83.33%
	PD2	2	443	21	12	92.68%
	PD2.5	0	36	69	3	63.89%
	PD3	0	29	2	77	71.30%
Precision		93.75%	86.19%	75.00%	83.70%	Accuracy 84.79%

Table 14.5 Discriminant results for subjects

		Predict					Recall
		PD1	PD2	PD2.5	PD3	Unknown	
Actual	PD1	1	0	0	0	0	100%
	PD2	0	13	0	0	0	100%
	PD2.5	0	1	2	0	0	66.67%
	PD3	0	1	0	2	0	66.67%
Precision		100%	86.67%	100%	100%	–	Accuracy 90%

classification performance for each utterance was 0.994 for sensitivity, 0.917 for specificity, and 0.952 for accuracy. Furthermore, the classification performance of each subject by the majority vote for each utterance result was 1.00, 1.00, and 1.00, respectively. Thus, the algorithm showed excellent performance in classifying healthy subjects and patients with Parkinson's disease, suggesting that it is useful for estimating the disease status based on utterances.

Conversely, in the voice index for discriminating the severity of Parkinson's disease, features that were considered effective for discrimination were selected in advance, and one of the features with a high correlation among the selected features was deleted. In feature selection, the discriminative performance of a single feature in the Parkinson's disease severity group was calculated by AUC, and the features that showed an AUC above a certain threshold for all combinations of the two groups (PD1 vs. PD2, PD1 vs. PD2.5, …, PD2.5 vs. PD3) were selected. Regularized multinomial logistic regression analysis (Friedman et al. 2010) was applied, using the remaining features as explanatory variables.

Consequently, a multigroup discriminant index consisting of 17 speech features was obtained. Table 14.4 shows the results of discriminating speech data using the multigroup discriminant index. The overall accuracy rate was approximately 85%. The stage prediction for each patient was based on the results of each speech. That is, the stage was predicted from each of the speech data for one examinee using the multigroup discriminant index, and the stage with the highest predictions was predicted as the examinee's stage. If the most frequently predicted stage was two or more, it was judged to be unknown. The results are presented in Table 14.5. Overall, an accuracy of 90% was obtained.

14.5 Discussion and Conclusions

In this study, we first examined a method that discriminated between PWPD and healthy individuals. These results suggest that PDVI is effective for screening for PWPD. However, the PDVI has not been validated in patient voices obtained from other hospitals. It is necessary to verify whether the coefficients introduced in Equation (14.1) can be used in the same manner. PDVI is similar to ALVI1, which is introduced in Chap. 7; PDVI is effective for screening PWPD, and ALVI is effective for screening patients with depression. Future studies are needed to verify whether PDVI is higher only in patients with Parkinson's disease or whether it is higher in patients with other diseases, such as depression than in normal subjects.

$$\mathrm{PDVI} = \mathrm{ZCR} + 0.23\mathrm{HE} - 0.215 \tag{14.1}$$

We also examined the methods to determine the severity of PWPD. These results suggest that it is possible to discriminate the severity of Parkinson's disease from speech. We used read speech rather than long vowel-like steady speech, and we expect that free speech will be used for detection in the future. However, because only one patient belonged to the PD1 group in the data used in this study, the discrimination of PD1 reflected only the characteristics of that patient, and the accuracy may not be sufficient for other data. Therefore, it is necessary to improve the accuracy of the index by validating it with other data or acquiring new patient data.

References

Bachu R, Kopparthi S, Adapa B, Barkana B (2010) Voiced/unvoiced decision for speech signals based on zero-crossing rate and energy. In: Elleithy K (ed) Advanced techniques in computing sciences and software engineering. Springer, Dordrecht, pp 279–282

Eom C, Choi S, Oh G, Jung WS (2008) Hurst exponent and prediction based on weak-form efficient market hypothesis of stock markets. Physica A 387:4630–4636

Eyben F, Wöllmer M, Schuller B (2010) openSMILE—The Munich Versatile and fast open-source audio feature extractor. In: Proceedings of the 18th ACM international conference on Multimedia, Firenze, 25-29 October 2010, pp 1459–1462

Friedman J, Hastie T, Tibshirani R (2010) Regularization paths for generalized linear models via coordinate descent. J Stat Softw 33(1):1–22

Jalil M, Butt FA, Malik A (2013) Short-time energy, magnitude, zero-crossing rate and autocorrelation measurement for discriminating voiced and unvoiced segments of speech signals. In Proceedings of the 2013 international conference on technological advances in electrical, electronics and computer engineering (TAEECE), Konya, Turkey, 9–11 May 2013, pp 208–212

Kazi MH, Ekramul H, Khademul IMA (2017) Method for voiced/unvoiced classification of noisy speech by analyzing time-domain features of spectrogram image. Sci J Circuits Syst Signal Process 6:11–17

Chapter 15
Dementia

Masakazu Higuchi

15.1 Introduction

The prevalence of dementia is increasing due to the aging of the population worldwide; the proportion of people aged 65 years or older is expected to be approximately 16% of the world population by 2050. It is estimated that approximately 100 million people will suffer from dementia (Prince et al. 2013; United Nations Population Division 2002). Therefore, the social cost of dementia is increasing annually, and early detection and preventive treatment are challenging.

In the early stages of dementia, it is difficult to differentiate it from depression and other disorders, and multiple tests are required to make a decision. Therefore, a simple initial screening method for dementia is needed. In clinical practice, neuropsychological tests are commonly used to screen for dementia, including the Mini-Mental State Examination (MMSE) (Folstein et al. 1975) and Mini-Cog (Borson et al. 2003). However, they must be performed by professionals and are not easy to use. Computed tomography (CT), magnetic resonance imaging (MRI), and positron emission tomography (PET) are also used for diagnostic imaging with relatively high accuracy; however, they are costly and invasive.

Our proposed voice-based diagnosis has thus far achieved a highly accurate detection of depression and Parkinson's disease. Therefore, we assumed that dementia also has an effect on voice and attempted to detect it using voice.

M. Higuchi (✉)
Department of Bioengineering, Graduate School of Engineering, The University of Tokyo, Bunkyo-ku, Tokyo, Japan
e-mail: higuchi@bioeng.t.u-tokyo.ac.jp

S. Tokuno, H. Nakamura (eds.), *Voice Biomarkers*,
https://doi.org/10.1007/978-981-96-3109-4_15

15.2 Detection of Dementia

Dementia can be broadly classified into Alzheimer's disease, Lewy body dementia, and cerebrovascular dementia (American Psychiatric Association 2000). We first examined whether we could identify patients diagnosed with dementia based on their voices without considering the type of dementia (Nakamura et al. 2018; Omiya et al. 2018; Tokuno 2020).

Nakamura et al. studied 37 patients (16 men and 21 women) diagnosed with dementia by physicians (Nakamura et al. 2018; Tokuno 2020). The voices of reading out fixed Japanese phrases, long vowels, and repeating pa-ta-ka were recorded in a hospital examination room using Portable Recorder R-26 (Roland, Japan). The recording format was 24-bit at 96 kHz. Additionally, a cognitive function test using the MMSE was performed by a physician. In this study, MMSE scores were estimated from the patients' voice features. The free software openSMILE version 2.3 (Eyben et al. 2010) was used to extract features from voice, and the feature set used in emotion recognition (the large openSMILE emotion feature set) was used to calculate 6552 voice features per utterance. They were (a) physical and similar features calculated frame by frame from a single voice: 56 types (fast Fourier transform, mel-frequency cepstral coefficient, voice probability, zero crossing rate, energy, fundamental frequency, etc.); (b) temporal processing of (a): 3 types (moving average, time variation (difference), time variation of time variation); and (c) statistical quantities for each type of (b): 39 types (mean, maximum, minimum, center of gravity, quartile, variance, kurtosis, skewness, etc.), for a total of $56 \times 3 \times 39 = 6552$ voice features. Correlation values with the MMSE scores were calculated for each feature. For each feature data, we divided the subjects into a group of subjects with an MMSE score of 24 or higher and a group of subjects with an MMSE score of less than 24; the feature means between the two groups were compared using a t-test to calculate the significance probability and effect size. A 24 MMSE score is the cut-off value for whether the subject has dementia. Feature values that were likely to be effective for MMSE score estimation were preselected using the above correlation values, significance probabilities, and effect sizes. Multiple regression analysis was conducted using the selected feature values as explanatory variables and the actual MMSE score as the objective variable. Among the regression coefficients obtained from the multiple regression analysis, the features for significant coefficients were selected, and the predicted values of the MMSE score were calculated using the prediction formula constructed from them. Multiple regression analysis was then conducted again, using the selected features as new explanatory variables and the predicted MMSE score as a new objective variable. Multiple regression analysis was repeated until all the regression coefficients were significant.

The analysis yielded a prediction formula comprising 11 features. The correlation value between the MMSE score calculated using the prediction formula and the actual MMSE score was approximately 0.7. Figure 15.1 shows a scatter plot. The receiver operating characteristic (ROC) curve for the MMSE prediction score when subjects with MMSE scores less than 24 were considered positive is shown in

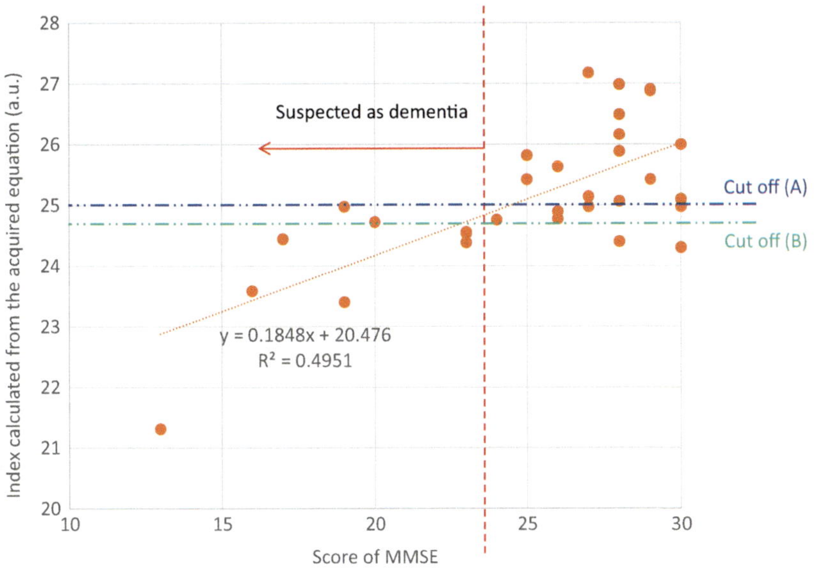

Fig. 15.1 Scatterplot of actual and predicted MMSE scores

Fig. 15.2 ROC curve for MMSE prediction score

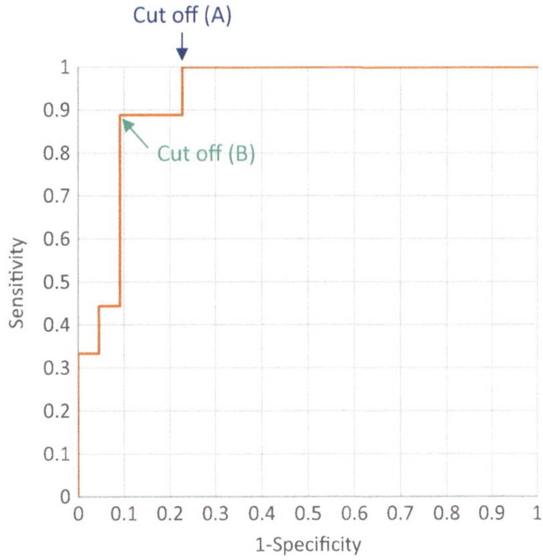

Fig. 15.2. The area under the ROC curve (AUC) was 0.88. The cut-off (B) in Fig. 15.1 is the best cut-off value for the MMSE prediction score, which is close to the actual MMSE score cut-off value for dementia. These results suggest that it is possible to estimate MMSE scores from voice.

Omiya et al. discriminated between patients with dementia and healthy individuals based on voice features in 39 patients (10 men and 29 women) diagnosed with

Table 15.1 Discrimination results for utterance data of dementia patients and healthy individuals

		Predicted group		
		Healthy	Dementia	Recall
Actual group	Healthy	344	133	0.721
	Dementia	134	949	0.876
	Precision	0.720	0.877	Accuracy 82.9%

dementia by a physician and in 18 healthy individuals (6 men and 12 women) who were living their daily lives without problems (Omiya et al. 2018). Voice recordings of fixed Japanese phrases were recorded in a hospital examination room using a Portable Recorder R-26 (Roland, Japan) in 24-bit and 96 kHz formats. The free software openSMILE version 2.3 was used to extract features from the voice, and 600 features derived from fast Fourier transform power, fundamental frequency, mel-frequency cepstrum coefficient, zero crossover rate, etc. were calculated from a single voice. Based on these features, a decision tree based on C4.5 (Quinlan 1993) was created using ten-fold cross-validation.

Table 15.1 shows the results of discriminating the voice data using the decision tree. Because the decision tree was created from voice data in units of utterances, the evaluation was conducted for each utterance and not for each subject. Sensitivity, specificity, and accuracy were 0.876, 0.721, and 0.829, respectively. To adjust for the imbalance in the data, we used the synthetic minority over-sampling technique (Chawla et al. 2002) to generate pseudo-healthy voice data and reconstructed a decision tree from these data. The discrimination results obtained using the decision tree are presented in Table 15.2. Sensitivity, specificity, and accuracy were 0.842, 0.843, and 0.842, respectively, and their sensitivity and specificity were almost equal. These results suggest that it is possible to discriminate patients with dementia from healthy individuals based on their voices.

15.3 Detection of Mild Cognitive Impairment

Mild cognitive impairment (MCI) is suspected when the MMSE score ranges from 24 to 27. Nakamura et al. showed that MMSE scores can be accurately predicted from voice features, but the predictions in the MCI region were not different from those in the healthy region, indicating that it is difficult to detect MCI (Nakamura et al. 2018; Tokuno 2020). MCI is an early stage of dementia, and its detection is important because it leads to early detection.

Higuchi et al. discriminated healthy individuals from MCI subjects based on voice features in subjects aged 65 years or older (Higuchi et al. 2021). Forty-five subjects (25 men and 20 women) who were living their daily lives without any problems were tested by a physician for cognitive function using the MMSE. The subjects were divided into two groups: a normal group (MMSE score ≥ 28) and a group with suspected MCI ($24 \leq$ MMSE score < 28). Voice recordings of fixed Japanese

Table 15.2 Discrimination results for utterance data containing pseudo-healthy data

		Predicted group		
		Healthy	Dementia	Recall
Actual group	Healthy	804	150	0.843
	Dementia	171	912	0.842
	Precision	0.825	0.859	Accuracy 84.2%

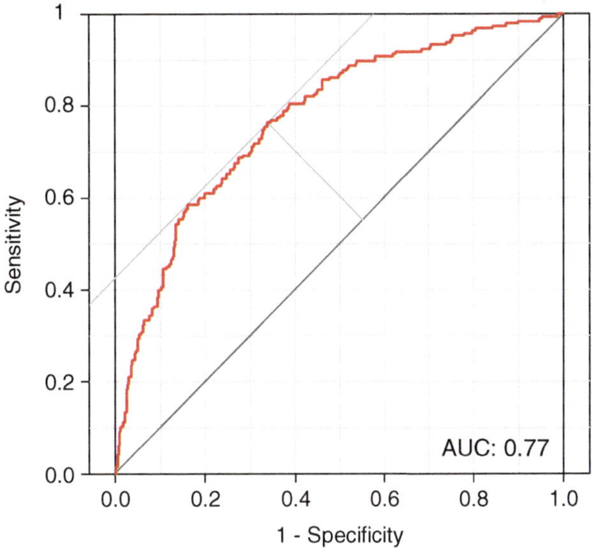

Fig. 15.3 ROC curve for predicted MCI

phrases were recorded in 24-bit and 96 kHz formats using Portable Recorder R-26 (Roland, Japan). The voice was divided into utterance units, and 6552 features of the large emotion feature set were calculated for each utterance using the free software openSMILE version 2.3. Regularized logistic regression analysis (Friedman et al. 2010) was applied to these features, and features with a cumulative contribution of up to 70% of the regression coefficients were selected.

Consequently, eight features were identified. The ROC curve for the predicted values of the utterance data calculated from the prediction formula consisting of these eight features is shown in Fig. 15.3, and the confusion matrix for the best cut-off value is shown in Table 15.3. The AUC was 0.77, and the sensitivity, specificity, and accuracy were 0.76, 0.66, and 0.69, respectively. The proportion of utterances discriminated as MCI was calculated for each subject based on the discrimination results of the utterance data, and predictions were made for each subject. The results are presented in Table 15.4. Sensitivity, specificity, and accuracy were 0.80, 0.77, and 0.78, respectively. The sensitivity, specificity, and accuracy for each subject were approximately 80%, suggesting the possibility of discriminating between MCI and healthy individuals from voice.

Table 15.3 Confusion matrix for the best cut-off value of MCI predictions

		Predicted group	
		Normal	MCI
Actual group	Normal	258	132
	MCI	47	148

Table 15.4 Discrimination result for each subject

		Predicted group	
		Normal	MCI
Actual group	Normal	23	7
	MCI	3	12

The study by Higuchi et al. showed only the prediction accuracy for training data, which may not be sufficient for unknown data. However, it has been reported that dual tasks, in which two tasks are performed simultaneously, are effective for detecting dementia. We focused on this point and hypothesized that, as cognitive function declines, task execution becomes more difficult, and the voice during task execution becomes significantly different from the normal voice. Based on this assumption, Nakamura et al. attempted to discriminate MCI from voice during task execution and proposed a data-independent index (Nakamura et al. 2022).

In this study, elderly people aged 60 years or older were recruited at two facilities, A and B, and requested to perform a calculation that continued to subtract 7 from 100, and the voice of the calculation was acquired. In addition to the calculated voice, the reading voice of a numerical value sequence was also acquired. The numerical sequences were 93, 86, 79, 72, and 65, respectively. This is the answer to the calculation by subtracting 7 from 100. Voice was recorded in the conference rooms of each facility using a Portable Recorder R-26 (Roland, Japan) in 24-bit and 96 kHz formats. Participants were also tested for cognitive ability using the MMSE and were divided into two groups at each facility: a normal group (MMSE score ≥ 28) and an MCI (suspected) group ($24 \leq$ MMSE score < 28). There were 199 participants in facility A and 20 participants in facility B. Large emotion feature sets were calculated using the free software openSMILE version 2.3. To eliminate individual differences, the features from the numerical string voice were considered as the base, and the amount of change from the base (the difference between the numerical string voice features and calculated voice features) was calculated. Thereafter, a decision tree was created using XGBoost (Chen and Guestrin 2016) with the amount of change in the features of facility A as the explanatory variable. The accuracy of the decision tree was verified using the feature value change of facility B.

The discriminant performance of the decision tree obtained using the ROC curve is shown in Fig. 15.4. Figure 15.4a shows the discrimination performance for facility A, and (b) shows the discrimination performance for facility B. For the data from facility A, the normal group and the MCI group were discriminated with 100% accuracy. For the data from facility B, which was not involved in the derivation of

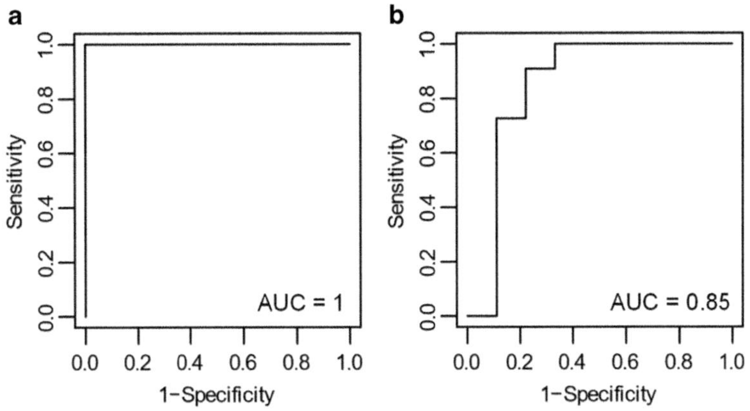

Fig. 15.4 (**a**) ROC curve for facility A and (**b**) ROC curve for facility B

the decision tree, an AUC of 0.85 was obtained, indicating a reasonable discrimination performance. Therefore, as we hypothesized, it was demonstrated that the voice was significantly different between task execution and normal times as cognitive function declined, and we proposed an index that is independent of the data. In this study, voice during single-task execution was used, and from this result, it can be expected that the voice during dual-task execution has a larger difference from the normal time than that during single-task execution. Future work will focus on discrimination using voice during dual-task executions.

15.4 Detection of Alzheimer's Disease

Because the possibility of voice-based diagnosis was suggested to some extent in the large framework of dementia, we next set out to study the individual types of dementia. First, we dealt with Alzheimer's disease (Omiya et al. 2019a, b, 2020, 2021).

Omiya et al. discriminated between healthy individuals and patients with Alzheimer's disease based on voice features in 57 healthy individuals (28 men and 29 women) who were living their daily lives without problems and in 42 patients (16 men and 26 women) who were diagnosed with Alzheimer's disease by their doctors at 6 hospitals (Omiya et al. 2019a, b). Voice recordings were made in the hospital examination rooms using a Portable Recorder R-26 (Roland, Japan). Voice recordings of fixed Japanese phrases were recorded in 24-bit and 96 kHz formats. Features were extracted from the voice using the free software openSMILE version 2.3, and 7440 features were calculated from a single utterance, including the large emotion feature set, features related to frequency bands not covered by the large emotion feature set, and features derived from them. To eliminate differences in recording environments between hospitals, differences between hospitals were evaluated for each feature in the healthy individuals and patients by testing, and features with significant differences were excluded. As a result, 197 features remained, and a decision tree based on C4.5 was created from these features using ten-fold cross-validation.

Table 15.5 shows the results of discriminating the voice data using the decision tree. Sensitivity, specificity, and accuracy were 0.697, 0.780, and 0.745, respectively, in the evaluation of the utterance units. The sensitivity and specificity were < 70% and > 70%, respectively, indicating a certain degree of discrimination accuracy.

Next, the 197-feature data were divided into 2 groups: 1 data group of 3 hospitals and the other data group of another 3 hospitals. One of the data groups was used as training data to reconstruct the decision tree. The accuracy of the reconstructed decision tree was validated for the other data groups. The validation results are presented in Table 15.6. Sensitivity, specificity, and accuracy were 0.513, 0.689, and 0.625, respectively. Furthermore, the decision tree was evaluated subject by subject. The predictions for each subject are based on the results of each utterance. For one subject, each utterance data was predicted by the decision tree, and the most predicted healthy and Alzheimer's disease was used as the prediction result of that subject. The results are presented in Table 15.7. Sensitivity, specificity, and accuracy were 0.591, 0.946, and 0.814, respectively. Sensitivity was not high for each utterance or subject. Specificity was much higher for each subject than for each utterance. As suggested by the results of the evaluation of the decision tree from the entire dataset (Table 15.5), the decision tree tended to fit healthy individuals better in the data used in this study. Although it is unclear why the decision tree did not fit the patients, the sensitivity of the decision tree was less than 70% for the entire dataset and less than 60% for each subject in the validation data, suggesting the possibility of discriminating Alzheimer's patients from healthy individuals, although the accuracy was not necessarily good.

Omiya et al. also examined the association between sound intensity-related features and Alzheimer's disease (Omiya et al. 2020). In severe Alzheimer's disease, physical ability declines to the point where it interferes with daily life. The decline in physical ability also weakens the ability to vibrate the vocal cords, which affects the voice. This effect is thought to extend to the strength of voice. This study included 20 healthy individuals who were living their daily lives without problems (HE) and 20 patients who had been diagnosed with Alzheimer's disease (AD) by their physicians. Because Parkinson's disease also causes a decline in physical

Table 15.5 Discrimination results for utterance of Alzheimer's disease patients and healthy individuals

		Predicted group		
		Healthy	Alzheimer's disease	Recall
Actual group	Healthy	1457	411	0.780
	Alzheimer's disease	421	970	0.697
	Precision	0.776	0.702	Accuracy 74.5%

Table 15.6 Discrimination results for utterances of Alzheimer's disease patients and healthy individuals in the validation group

		Predicted group		
		Healthy	Alzheimer's disease	Recall
Actual group	Healthy	887	400	0.689
	Alzheimer's disease	359	378	0.513
	Precision	0.712	0.486	Accuracy 62.5%

Table 15.7 Discrimination results for Alzheimer's disease patients and healthy individuals in the validation group

		Predicted group		
		Healthy	Alzheimer's disease	Recall
Actual group	Healthy	35	2	0.946
	Alzheimer's disease	9	13	0.591
	Precision	0.796	0.867	Accuracy 81.4%

ability, 20 patients diagnosed by a physician with Parkinson's disease (PD) were also included for comparison. Voice recordings were made in the hospital examination room using a Portable Recorder R-26 (Roland, Japan). The voice of repeating pa-ta-ka for 5 s was recorded in 24-bit and 96 kHz formats. As features related to sound intensity, we calculated (1) the slope of sound intensity; (2) the mean, (3) the standard deviation, and (4) the slope of the peak value of sound intensity; and (5) the mean and (6) the standard deviation of the peak interval. For each of these six features, the mean values in the HE, AD, and PD groups were compared using the Tukey–Kramer test (Tukey 1949).

As a result, significant differences were found between the HE and PD groups in (3) and between the HE and AD groups and between the AD and PD groups in (5). The distribution of each feature for each group is shown in Fig. 15.5. Although Alzheimer's and Parkinson's diseases had similar symptoms, there tended to be differences in the distribution of the features that were considered to be relevant to both diseases. These results suggest that sound intensity can be used to discriminate between healthy individuals, patients with Alzheimer's disease, and patients with Parkinson's disease.

Omiya et al. further confirmed the trend shown in Omiya et al. (2020) for another dataset (Omiya et al. 2021). This study included 23 healthy individuals, 22 patients with Alzheimer's disease, and 20 patients with Parkinson's disease. Voice data were pre-normalized to reduce differences in the recording environment. Furthermore, in this study, the median sound intensity was used as a threshold for detecting the peak sound intensity values, and peak values above the threshold were detected to avoid detecting outliers as much as possible. In addition, the new peak value was defined as the maximum value within 0.1 s from the time of the previous peak value.

Figure 15.6 shows the results of the Tukey–Kramer test comparing the mean values of features (1) to (6) in the HE, AD, and PD groups. Compared to Omiya et al. (2021), (1), (2), (5), and (6) showed similar trends. Significant differences

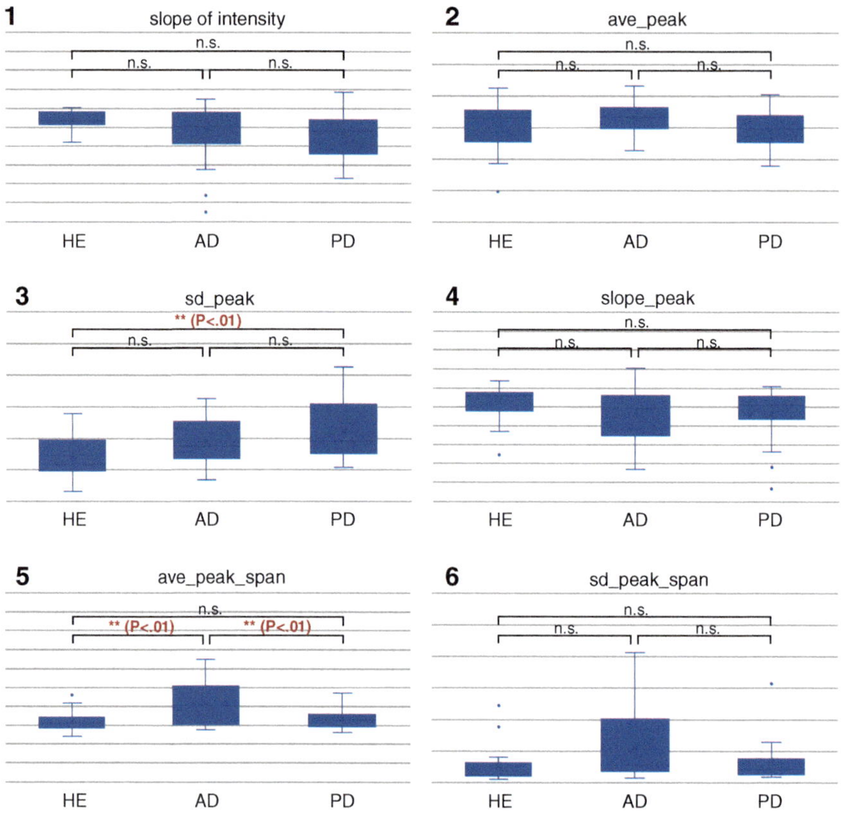

Fig 15.5 Distribution of features related to sound intensity for HE, AD, and PD groups

were confirmed in at least one combination of two groups from the HE, AD, and PD groups for features other than (2). Therefore, the possibility that sound intensity can be used to discriminate between healthy individuals, patients with Alzheimer's disease, and patients with Parkinson's disease was confirmed.

Decreased physical ability also occurs in patients with dementia and Lewy bodies. Future work should include voice data from patients with dementia and Lewy bodies for comparison with patients with Alzheimer's disease.

15.5 Detection of Dementia with Lewy Bodies

We next embarked on a study on dementia with Lewy bodies. Dementia with Lewy bodies is said to be more hypersensitive to medications and more prone to immediate side effects than Alzheimer's disease, and inappropriate medication dosages often lead to a diagnosis of this disease as the disease worsens (American Psychiatric

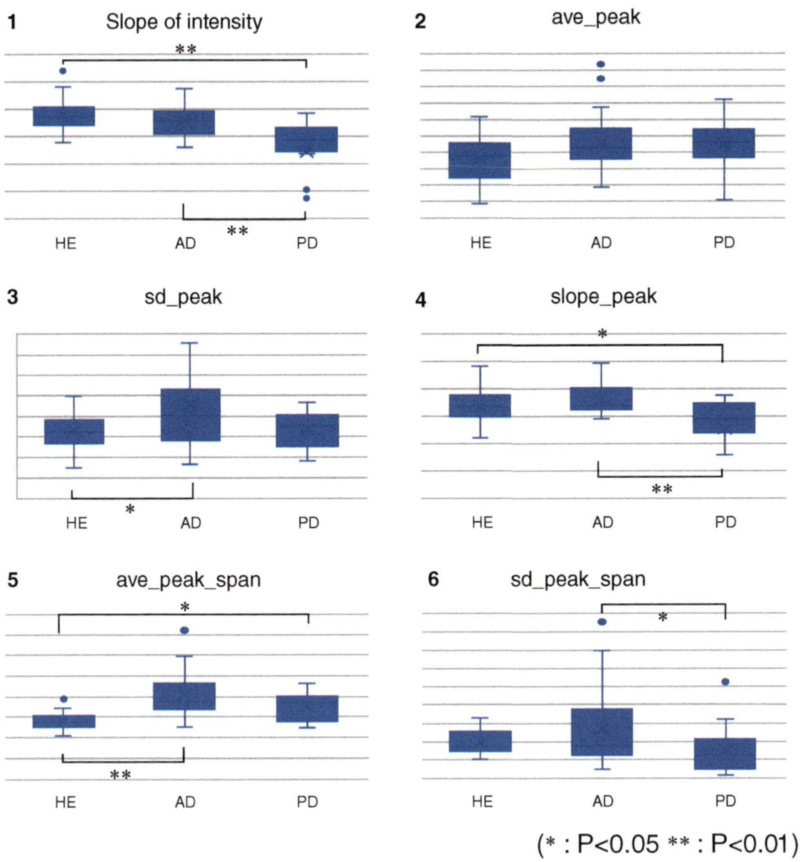

Fig. 15.6 Distribution of features related to sound intensity for HE, AD, and PD groups

Association 2000). Therefore, we considered that the early detection of the disease by voice diagnosis would prevent the use of inappropriate doses of medication.

Omiya et al. discriminated between healthy individuals and patients with dementia with Lewy bodies based on voice features in 20 healthy individuals (6 men and 14 women) who were living their daily lives without problems and in 20 patients (8 men and 12 women) who were diagnosed with dementia with Lewy bodies (DLB) by their doctors at 3 hospitals (Omiya et al. 2019c). Voice recordings were made in the hospital examination rooms using a Portable Recorder R-26 (Roland, Japan). Voices of fixed Japanese phrases were recorded in 24-bit and 96 kHz formats. The free software openSMILE version 2.3 was used to extract features from the voice, and 6552 features of the large emotion feature set were calculated per voice. To eliminate differences in recording environments between hospitals, differences between hospitals of each feature were evaluated by testing in healthy individuals and patients, and features with significant differences were excluded. Consequently, 168 features remained. Furthermore, the mean values of these features were

Table 15.8 Discriminant results for validation data of utterance unit

		Predicted group		
		Healthy	DLB	Recall
Actual group	Healthy	40	13	0.755
	DLB	13	38	0.745
	Precision	0.755	0.745	Accuracy 75.0%

compared between the healthy and DLB groups using a test, and features that were significantly different between the two groups were selected. Consequently, 16 features were identified. Based on these features, a decision tree was created using the LightGBM (Guolin et al. 2017). The decision tree was created using five-fold cross-validation with 90% of the feature data as training data. The remaining 10% of the feature data were then used to validate the decision tree.

The discrimination results are shown in Table 15.8. Sensitivity, specificity, and accuracy were 0.755, 0.745, and 0.750, respectively. The sensitivity, specificity, and accuracy were all > 70%, suggesting that it is possible to discriminate patients with Lewy body dementia from healthy individuals.

15.6 Conclusion

We investigated whether it was possible to discriminate dementia from voice disorders. First, voice discrimination may be effective in the broad framework of dementia. However, because the discrimination accuracy was not sufficient for MCI, we focused on MCI and attempted to discriminate it from voice. We discriminated MCI with a certain degree of accuracy. Next, we focused on the types of dementia. The sensitivity of the voice-based discriminant for Alzheimer's disease was insufficient, but good sensitivity was obtained for dementia with Lewy bodies. We also compared the distribution of voice features in Alzheimer's disease and Parkinson's disease, assuming that voice features are affected by symptoms common to both diseases. The results suggested that the distributions of voice features tended to differ between Alzheimer's disease and Parkinson's disease. Therefore, the possibility that Alzheimer's disease and Parkinson's disease can be differentiated by voice has been demonstrated.

Based on the above results, it was concluded that it is possible to discriminate dementia from voice, to some extent. For future studies, it is necessary to verify various data groups for the differentiation of Alzheimer's and Lewy body dementia, discrimination of dementia, depression, and Parkinson's disease and to improve the accuracy of MCI discrimination.

References

American Psychiatric Association (2000) Diagnostic and statistical manual of mental disorders, 4th edn, text revision. American Psychiatric Publications Inc., New York

Borson S, Scanlan JM, Chen P, Ganguli M (2003) The Mini-Cog as a screen for dementia: validation in a population-based sample. J Am Geriatr Soc 51(10):1451–1454

Chawla NV, Bowyer KW, Hall LO, Kegelmeyer WP (2002) SMOTE: synthetic minority over-sampling technique. J Artif Intell Res 16:321–357

Chen T, Guestrin C (2016) XGBoost: a scalable tree boosting system. In: Proceedings of the 22nd ACM SIGKDD international conference on knowledge discovery and data mining (KDD2016), California, 13–17 August 2016

Eyben F, Wöllmer M, Schuller B (2010) openSMILE—The Munich Versatile and fast open-source audio feature extractor. In: Proceedings of the 18th ACM international conference on Multimedia, Firenze, 25–29 October 2010, pp 1459–1462

Folstein MF, Folstein SE, McHugh PR (1975) "Mini-mental state". A practical method for grading the cognitive state of patients for the clinician. J Psychiatr Res 12:189–198

Friedman J, Hastie T, Tibshirani R (2010) Regularization paths for generalized linear models via coordinate descent. J Stat Softw 33(1):1–22

Guolin K, Qi M, Thomas F, Taifeng W, Wei C, Weidong M, Qiwei Y, Tie-Yan L (2017) LightGBM: a highly efficient gradient boosting decision tree. In: Proceedings of the 31st international conference on neural information processing systems (NIPS2017), California, 4–9 December 2017

Higuchi M, Nakamura M, Okazaki T, Takemura J, Takano T, Omiya Y, Shinohara S, Mitsuyoshi S, Tokuno S (2021) Detection of mild cognitive impairment by voice [Translated from Japanese]. In: Abstracts of the 60th annual conference of Japanese Society for Medical and Biological Engineering, Virtual, 15–17 June 2021 (in Japanese)

Nakamura M, Shinohara S, Omiya Y, Higuchi M, Hagiwara N, Takano T, Mitsuyoshi S, Nozaki Y, Yoshitake M, Sanjo N, Tokuno S (2018) Feasibility study on screening for dementia using voice analysis. In: Abstracts of the 40th international engineering in medicine and biology conference (EMBC2018), Hawaii, 17–21 July 2018

Nakamura M, Higuchi M, Omiya Y, Takano T, Shinohara T, Mitsuyoshi S, Tokuno S (2022) Detection of mild cognitive impairment using difference of voice features between conditions. In: Abstracts of the 16th international conference on Alzheimer's and Parkinson's diseases (AD/PD 2022), Virtual, 15–20 March 2022

Omiya Y, Takano T, Uraguchi T, Nakamura M, Shinohara S, Higuchi M, Mitsuyoshi S, Tokuno S (2018) Pilot study to detect Dementia based on vocal analysis. In: Abstracts of neuroscience 2018, San Diego, 3–7 November 2018

Omiya Y, Nakamura M, Shinohara S, Higuchi M, Takano T, Uraguchi T, Mitsuyoshi S, Ishida M, Sanjo S, Tokuno S (2019a) Pilot study to detect Alzheimer's disease based on vocal analysis. In: Abstracts of the 14th international conference on Alzheimer's and Parkinson's diseases (AD/PD2019), Lisbon, 26–31 March 2019

Omiya Y, Nakamura M, Shinohara S, Higuchi M, Takano T, Uraguchi T, Mitsuyoshi S, Sanjo N, Tokuno S (2019b) A study on detection of Alzheimer's disease based on voice analysis [Translated from Japanese]. In: Abstracts of the 58th annual conference of Japanese Society for Medical and Biological Engineering, Okinawa, 6–8 June 2019 (in Japanese)

Omiya Y, Uraguchi T, Takano T, Nakamura M, Shinohara S, Higuchi M, Suzuki K, Manome N, Ishida M, Kumamoto Y, Mitsuyoshi S, Tokuno S (2019c) Pilot study of distinguishing between dementia with Lewy bodies and healthy subjects using voice. In: Abstracts of neuroscience 2019, Chicago, 19–23 October 2019

Omiya Y, Takano T, Uraguchi T, Nakamura M, Higuchi M, Shinohara S, Mitsuyoshi S, Ishida M, Kumamoto Y, Tokuno S (2020) A pilot study to distinguish between healthy participant and patient with Alzheimer's disease and Parkinson's disease based on vocal analysis. In: Abstracts of advances in Alzheimer's and Parkinson's therapies (AAT-AD/PD2020), Virtual, 2–5 April 2020

Omiya Y, Takano T, Higuchi M, Nakamura M, Shinohara S, Mitsuyoshi S, Sanjo N, Terashi H, Tokuno S (2021) A pilot study to distinguish between healthy participant and patient with Alzheimer's disease and Parkinson's disease based on vocal analysis: follow-up report. In: Abstracts of the 15th international conference on Alzheimer's and Parkinson's diseases (AD/PD 2021), Virtual, 9–14 March 2021

Prince M, Guerchet M, Prina M (2013) The global impact of dementia 2013–2050. Alzheimer's Disease International, London

Quinlan JR (1993) C4.5: programs for machine learning. Morgan Kaufmann Publishers, New York

Tokuno S (2020) Ageing: detection of cognitive impairment using voice analysis technology. Open Access Govern 2020(4):256–257

Tukey JW (1949) Comparing individual means in the analysis of variance. Biometrics 5(2):99–114

United Nations Population Division (2002) World population ageing: 1950–2050. Global Action on Aging, New York

Chapter 16
Differential Diagnosis

Shinichi Tokuno

16.1 Introduction

The US Food and Drug Administration (FDA) classifies biomarkers into diagnostic, monitoring, response, predictive, prognostic, safety, and susceptibility/risk biomarkers and reasonably likely surrogate endpoints (FDA 2016). For voice biomarkers, what is important is their use as diagnostic, monitoring, or response biomarkers. In other words, voice-based screening can be used to detect (diagnose) diseases at an early stage, monitor disease progression and remission, and confirm the response to and efficacy of drug therapies and other interventions.

Time-series or longitudinal searches, such as monitoring or determining the efficacy of a treatment for an already diagnosed disease, i.e., monitoring or response biomarkers, are possible by capturing the differences between healthy subjects and the disease. However, when considering using a biomarker as a diagnostic biomarker (e.g., a cross-sectional search for screening and other purposes), a comparison with healthy subjects is insufficient. Of course, a physician's diagnosis is not based on a single biomarker alone but rather comprehensively on the results of many tests, including symptoms and biomarkers. Nonetheless, if a biomarker is used for screening, it cannot be used if it changes with too many diseases. In other words, biomarkers for screening must be developed with minimal false positives. Hence, differential diagnosis needs to be validated using voice.

S. Tokuno (✉)
Department of Bioengineering, Graduate School of Engineering, The University of Tokyo, Bunkyo-ku, Tokyo, Japan
e-mail: tokuno@bioeng.t.u-tokyo.ac.jp

S. Tokuno, H. Nakamura (eds.), *Voice Biomarkers*,
https://doi.org/10.1007/978-981-96-3109-4_16

16.2 Differential Diagnosis by Voice Biomarkers

Few studies on voice biomarkers have compared two or more diseases for differential diagnosis. Kowalska-Taczanowska et al. (2020) reported voice-related differences between Parkinson's disease and atypical Parkinsonism. Daoudi et al. (2021) reported that it was possible to differentiate Parkinson's disease from multiple system atrophy, which are considered to have similar initial symptoms, by voice. In the field of psychiatry, Shin et al. (2021) also reported that major and minor depressions could be differentiated by voice. Espinola et al. (2022) reported that voice could be used to differentiate between four categories of depression: major depression, bipolar disorder, schizophrenia, and anxiety disorders.

We have also noted that voice biomarkers can be altered in other diseases (Shinohara et al. 2017a, b). For example, Fig. 16.1 shows the differences in the MIMOSYS voice indices, between healthy subjects and patients with depression and poststroke dysarthria. The differences between normal subjects and patients with depression and poststroke dysarthria are clear, but no differences can be observed in patients with depression and poststroke dysarthria. Although poststroke patients show a tendency toward depression due to loss of function, this study could not clarify whether the decrease in the voice index after stroke is due to concomitant depressive symptoms or functional dysarthria. To clarify this, a different voice index is required to discriminate between dysarthria and depressive symptoms. If such an index were to exist, it would be possible to determine whether the decline in the MIMOSYS index in poststroke patients is due to depressive symptoms or dysarthria.

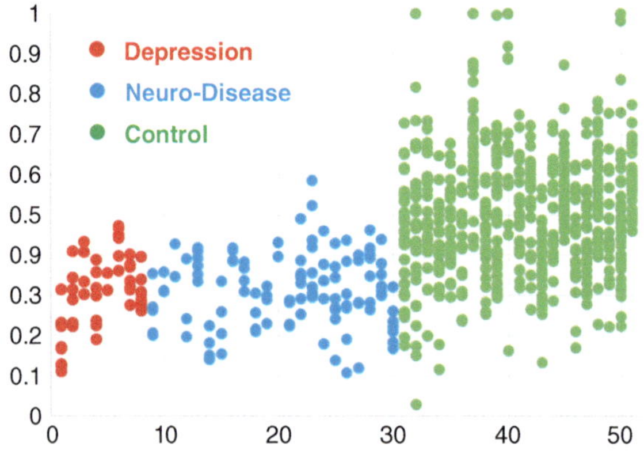

Fig. 16.1 Differentiation of depression and dysarthria by MIMOSYS. The differences between normal subjects and patients with depression and poststroke dysarthria are clear, but no differences can be observed in patients with depression and poststroke dysarthria

16.3 Parkinson's Disease, Depression, and Dementia

Despite the points raised above, however, it is not realistic to construct a system to differentiate all diseases, as this would require a large number of voice samples. Hence, we focused on areas in which there is the greatest need and worked on the development of diagnostic biomarkers. In other words, we selected three diseases: depression (in the elderly), dementia, and Parkinson's disease (Fig. 16.2). These three diseases are common in the elderly, have high comorbidity rates, and have similar symptoms in their early stages.

We attempted to differentiate Parkinson's disease from depression using the original features described in Chap. 7 and similar indices to those used for Parkinson's disease in Chap. 14, which are based on the zero crossing rate (ZCR) and Hurst exponent (HE). For depression, the voice signal was divided into small segments, and the ZCR and HE were calculated for each segment. A regression line was obtained from the ZCR and HE data for all segments, and the intercept of this line was used as the major depression voice index (MDVI). On the other hand, the index used in Chap. 8 (PDVI) was used for Parkinson's disease (Fig. 16.3).

Figure 16.4 shows the results of adaptation to 17 different standardized reading voices obtained from healthy subjects ($N = 32$), patients with major depression ($N = 25$), and patients with Parkinson's disease ($N = 15$). As shown in the figure, the MDVI responded to both major depression and Parkinson's disease, while the PDVI responded only to Parkinson's disease. The combination of both indices was shown to differentiate between the three categories of healthy, major depression, and Parkinson's disease (Shinohara et al. 2017a, b).

Another method for differential diagnosis is the validation of machine learning for differential diagnosis between Parkinson's disease and major depression. In this validation, the openSMILE software (Eyben et al. 2010) was used to extract 6552 acoustic features from individuals' voices; then, a healthy subject's voice was used to exclude features that could be classified according to environmental differences, such as recording location and season. Next, a J48 decision tree induction algorithm (Weka [Hall et al. 2009] implementation of C4.5) and 10-fold cross-validation were

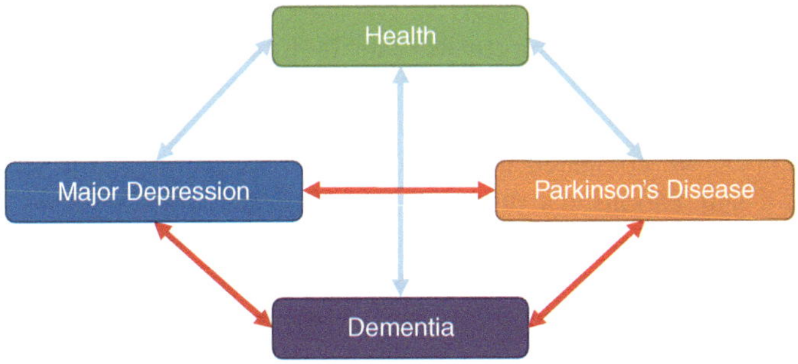

Fig. 16.2 Target diseases in differential diagnosis. We selected three diseases: depression (in the elderly), dementia, and Parkinson's disease

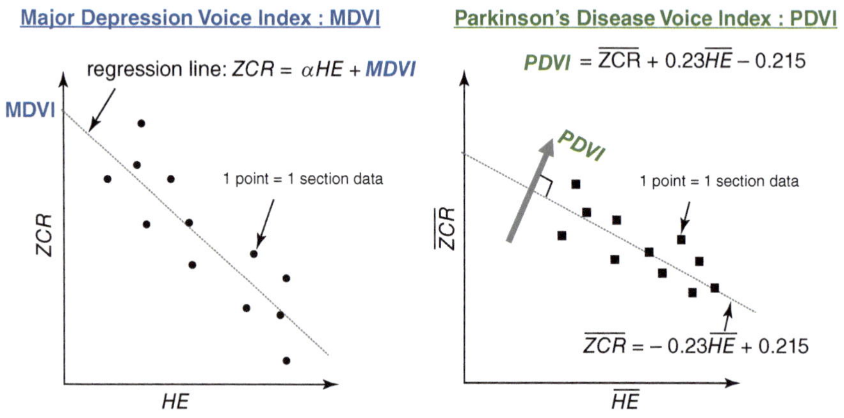

Fig. 16.3 MDVI and PDVI. See detail in Chap. 8

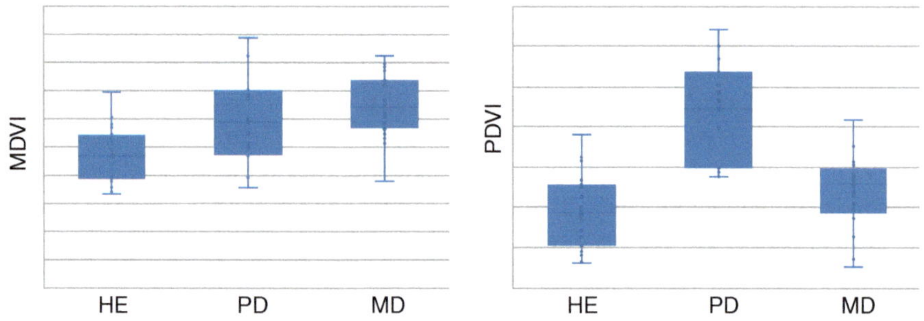

Fig. 16.4 Differentiation between Parkinson's disease and major depression by two voice indicators. *HE* healthy, *PD* Parkinson's disease, *MD* major depression

used to develop an algorithm to classify healthy subjects and patients with Parkinson's disease or major depression using 80 extracted features. As listed in Table 16.1, the classification performance of the algorithm relative to healthy subjects, patients with a major depression disease, and patients with Parkinson's disease was 75.9% with a recall of 0.781, 0.742, and 0.750, respectively, and precision of 0.676, 0.767, and 0.938, respectively. The algorithm successfully classified three categories: normal, Parkinson's disease, and major depression. Machine learning analysis of voice has been shown to be sufficient for differential diagnosis.

In Chap. 15, we compared the distribution of voice features with respect to Alzheimer's and Parkinson's diseases, assuming that voice features would be affected by symptoms common to both diseases. The results of the comparison between Alzheimer's disease and Parkinson's disease suggest that the distribution of voice features tends to differ between Alzheimer's disease and Parkinson's disease.

An algorithm for differentiating depression from dementia is currently under development and validation.

Table. 16.1 Classification matrix

		Classified		
		Healthy	**MD**[a]	**PD**[b]
Actual	**Healthy**	25	8	4
	MD[a]	6	23	1
	PD[b]	1	0	15

[a]*MD* major depression, [b]*PD* Parkinson's disease

16.4 Bipolar Disorder and Major Depression

Patients with bipolar disorder often first visit a clinic during the depressive phase. However, it is often difficult to immediately diagnose bipolar disorder because the patient is unaware that he or she is bipolar. In fact, it has been reported that 65% of patients with bipolar disorder were initially diagnosed with depression (Watanabe et al. 2016). If the voice at initial diagnosis suggests the possibility of bipolar disorder, this could lead to effective treatment.

As presented in Chap. 20, analyzing multiple voice features using logistic regression analysis, we were able to discriminate between healthy, bipolar, and major depressive disorder groups with high accuracy. Further validations in the future may reduce the number of patients with bipolar disorder being initially diagnosed with depression.

16.5 Summary

In this chapter, we showed that voice can be used to differentiate between three major similar illnesses in the elderly: depression, Parkinson's disease, and dementia. In contrast, voice cannot be used to differentiate between dementia and depression. Voice can also be used to differentiate between major depression and the depressive phase of bipolar disorder. These results indicate that voice biomarkers can function not only as monitoring or response biomarkers but also as diagnostic biomarkers.

References

Daoudi K, Das B, de Saint Victor SM, Foubert-Samier A, Pavy-Le Traon A et al (2021) Distortion of voiced obstruents for differential diagnosis between Parkinson's disease and multiple system atrophy. INTERSPEECH 2021

Eyben F, Wllmer M, Schuller B (2010) Opensmile: the Munich versatile and fast open-source audio feature extractor. In: Bimbo AD, Chang SF, Smeulders AWM (eds) ACM multimedia, pp 1459–1462

FDA-NIH Biomarker Working Group (2016) BEST (Biomarkers, EndpointS, and other Tools) resource. Food and Drug Administration/National Institutes of Health, Silver Spring/Bethesda www.ncbi.nlm.nih.gov/books/NBK326791/. Accessed 7 June 2022

Hall M, Frank E, Holmes G, Pfahringer B, Reutemann P, Witten IH (2009) The WEKA data mining software: an update. ACM SIGKDD Explor Newsl 11(1):10–18

Kowalska-Taczanowska R, Friedman A, Koziorowski D (2020) Parkinson's disease or atypical Parkinsonism? The importance of acoustic voice analysis in differential diagnosis of speech disorders. Brain Behav 10(8):e01700

Shin D, Cho WI, Park CHK, Rhee SJ, Kim MJ, Lee H et al (2021) Detection of minor and major depression through voice as a biomarker using machine learning. J Clin Med 10(14):3046

Shinohara S, Omiya Y, Hagiwara N, Nakamura M, Higuchi M, Kirita T, Takano T, Mitsuyoshi S, Tokuno S (2017a) Case studies of utilization of the mind monitoring system (MIMOSYS) using voice and its future prospects. ESMSJ (Econophys Sociophys Other Multidiscip Sci Jl) 7(1):7–12

Shinohara S, Omiya Y, Nakamura M, Higuchi M, Hagiwara N, Takano T, Mitsuyoshi S, Tokuno S (2017b) Identification of patients with Parkinson's disease, major depressed patients and healthy subjects by voice indices. IEICE Tech Rep. https://www.ieice.org/ken/paper/201712134byl/eng/

Wanderley Espinola C, Gomes JC, Mônica Silva Pereira J, dos Santos WP (2022) Detection of major depressive disorder, bipolar disorder, schizophrenia and generalized anxiety disorder using vocal acoustic analysis and machine learning: an exploratory study. Res Biomed Eng 38(3):813–829

Watanabe K, Harada E, Inoue T, Tanji Y, Kikuchi T (2016) Perceptions and impact of bipolar disorder in Japan: results of an Internet survey. Neuropsychiatr Dis Treat:2981–2987

Chapter 17
Sleep Apnea Syndrome

Mitsuteru Nakamura

17.1 Introduction

Sleep apnea syndrome (SAS) causes high-frequency hypopnea or apnea during sleep. Sleep quality deteriorates owing to the decreased sleep depth caused by hypopnea and apnea, which directly impacts sleep, resulting in a lack of substantial sleep relative to the amount of time spent asleep. This can lead to unintentional dozing during the daytime and cause accidents (Findley et al. 1998), and it has received significant social attention. In addition, the effects of hypoxia caused by hypopnea and apnea on body tissues (Ryan et al. 2005), and the strain on the cardiovascular system to recover from hypoxia increases the risk of lifestyle-related diseases, such as hypertension (Lavie et al. 2000), diabetes (Tasali et al. 2008), and even major depression (Sharafkhaneh et al. 2005).

There are two leading causes of SAS: obstructive SAS (OSA), caused by physical narrowing or obstruction of the airways, and central SAS, caused by problems with nerve signals from the brain related to respiratory motion. Because of the high percentage of patients with OSA, this study focused on OSA.

M. Nakamura (✉)
Department of Bioengineering, Graduate School of Engineering, The University of Tokyo, Bunkyo-ku, Tokyo, Japan
e-mail: nakamura@bioeng.t.u-tokyo.ac.jp

S. Tokuno, H. Nakamura (eds.), *Voice Biomarkers*,
https://doi.org/10.1007/978-981-96-3109-4_17

17.2 Evaluation of Sleep Quality and Treatment Effectiveness Against SAS Using Mood Index Before and After Sleep

Sleep quality may affect mood, as SAS is known to increase the risk of comorbid major depression.

A study was conducted to examine the relationship between the assessment of emotions using Sensibility Technology (ST) (Mitsuyoshi et al. 2006), a voice emotion analysis technology, and the assessment of mental health status using the General Health Questionnaire (Goldberg 1978), a self-administered questionnaire in a 30-question version (GHQ30) and its subscales. The results are shown in Fig. 17.1. One of the GHQ30 subscales, an index related to sleep disturbance, is significantly correlated with feelings of anger, suggesting that sleep disturbance may cause negative emotions.

Next, with the cooperation of the Minato Mirai Clinic (Yokohama, Japan), a clinic that conduct sleep tests, a study was conducted to evaluate the relationship between sleep-related data using polysomnography (PSG), the gold standard for SAS diagnosis, and voice-guided mental health indices. Participants were recruited among PSG patients at the clinic. While PSG provides a large amount of data, this study used the summary data provided in the reports notified to test-takers. Because snoring during sleep is an acoustic signal but not the same as speech and usual speech recording during PSG is unavailable, the participants were asked to read a

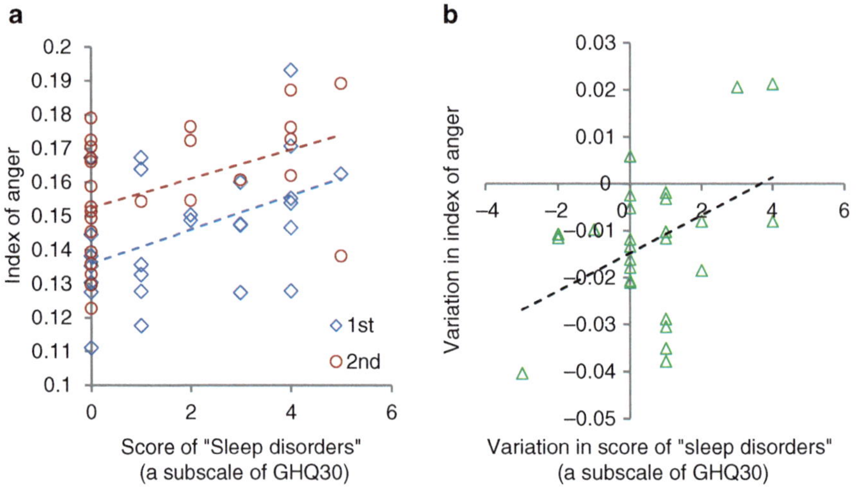

Fig. 17.1 Scatterplot between score of sleep disorders evaluated based on GHQ30 and intensity of anger emotion calculated using voice emotion analysis. Measurements were performed twice: the second measurement was conducted approximately 3 months after the first. (**a**) Samples in each measurement. (**b**) Variations in each index between two measurements. (Modified from Nakamura et al. 2015)

set text immediately before going to bed and immediately after waking. Their speeches were recorded and analyzed in this study.

In this study, many of the participants were possible SAS patients as they had some concern about their sleep. The most critical index of SAS obtained using PSG is the apnea–hypopnea index (AHI), calculated as the sum of the number of apnea and hypopnea events per hour. An AHI of five or higher indicates SAS, which can be further divided into three severity levels based on the AHI (Ruehland et al. 2009). In clinical practice in Japan, if the AHI is 20 or higher, continuous positive air pressure (CPAP), a symptomatic treatment method for SAS, is covered by public medical insurance in Japan. This criterion is considered the standard for patients with SAS requiring treatment. Usage of CPAP is decided by the will of the patient based on the recommendation by the clinic. At the beginning of CPAP treatment, a PSG test with using CPAP called titration (TR) is conducted to determine the CPAP operating parameters. However, if the AHI from the PSG test indicates that the patient has severe SAS, CPAP treatment is started before TR adjustment with the patient's consent. In this study, participants who provided consent were also audio-recorded immediately before bedtime and immediately after waking during TR. This was an observational study with no intervention and only a few recordings within the typical clinical protocol.

The recorded voices were analyzed using the MIMOSYS algorithm (Omiya et al. 2016), which calculates the overall measure of mental health based on the ratio of emotional indices obtained through voice emotion recognition (Mitsuyoshi et al. 2006). Because of the limited opportunities for voice recording in this study, mental activity, a long-term index obtained through continuous measurements, was not used; vitality, a short-term index obtained by a single measurement, was used as the main index instead of mental activity.

The working hypothesis was that vitality immediately after sleep is influenced by sleep quality. Because the intraindividual baseline of vitality may not be explained solely based on sleep, we also considered that the effect of sleep could be extracted by assuming that vitality immediately before sleep reflected the baseline and taking the difference in vitality before and after sleep and considering it as the amount of change.

Although some participants in this study did not receive CPAP treatment and only PSG data were collected, we analyzed only the data for participants who continued to participate in the study after TR for comparison. The timing of the recordings made by the participants included in the analysis is shown in Fig. 17.2. Among these participants, those who performed TR immediately before CPAP use were classified as Group A, and those who started CPAP use before TR was performed were categorized as Group B.

Figure 17.3 shows the distribution of vitality at each recording time point for each group. It was hypothesized that sleep quality of the participants during the first PSG was poor as they were SAS patients requiring CPAP treatment. The vitality at (2) tends to be lower than that at (1), indicating that sleep did not improve vitality but rather worsened it. This tendency infers that SAS impacted the sleep quality. However, statistical tests showed no significant differences. In addition, because

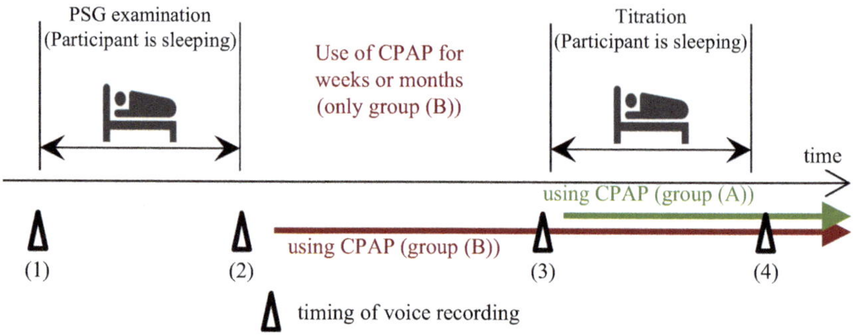

Fig. 17.2 Diagram for voice recording timings in this study. (1) Just before first PSG measurement; (2) just after first PSG measurement; (3) just after titration (second PSG using CPAP); (4) just after titration. (Modified from Nakamura et al. 2018)

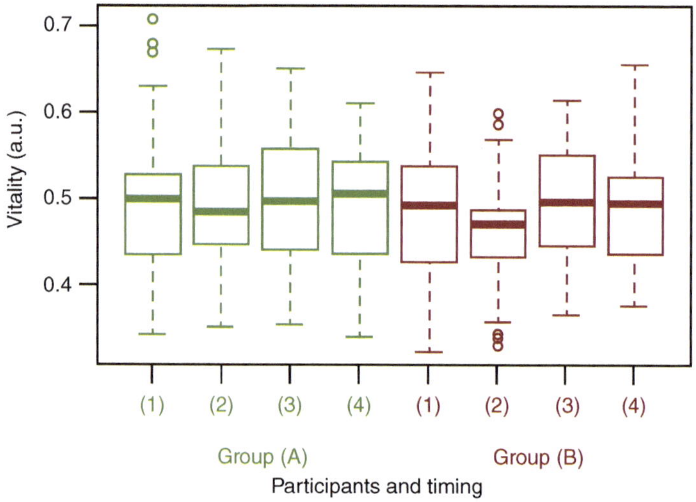

Fig. 17.3 Boxplot of vitality measured through voice analysis in each participant group and timing of measurement. Numbers on the horizontal axis show measurement timings described in Fig. 17.2. Left half shows the results in the participant group (**a**), and right half shows the results in the participant group (**b**). (Modified from Nakamura et al. 2018)

CPAP is used during TR, the therapeutic effect might be observed, and the decrease at (4) from (3) may be suppressed.

To clarify the impact of this change, the distributions of vitality change before and after PSG and TR, i.e., (2)–(1) and (4)–(3), respectively, were determined (Fig. 17.4). These differences can be summarized as the effect of sleep on restoring the overall health of the body and mind as measured using vitality. The effect of sleep in Fig. 17.4 is more apparent than in Fig. 17.3. Moreover, there is a tendency for the decline in vitality to be suppressed more during TR (4)–(3), when some form of treatment was provided, than during PSG (2)–(1), when SAS was untreated.

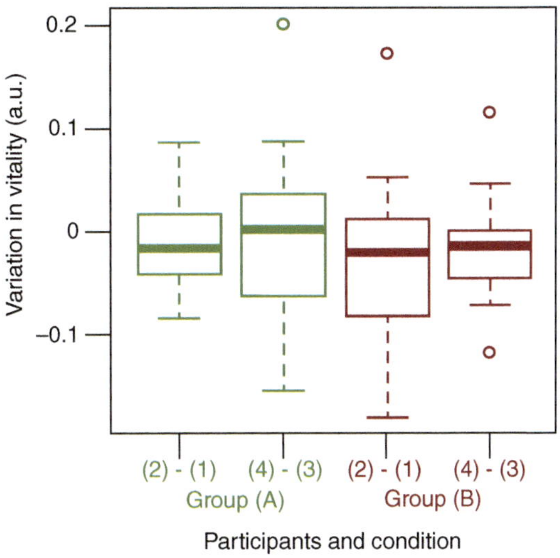

Fig. 17.4 Boxplot of variation in vitality between immediately before and after sleep. If the value is positive, the sleep yields a positive effect for the participant and vice versa. Left half shows the results in the participant group (**a**), and right half shows the results in the participant group (**b**). (Modified from Nakamura et al. 2018)

However, the statistical test could not determine whether a significant difference existed.

The reasons for these results might be that the participants in Group A used CPAP for the first time during TR, and the therapeutic effect of CPAP may not be optimal for all participants, as TR is a process of adjusting CPAP to a suitable condition for each patient. For the participants in Group B, at least 1 month had passed since they started using CPAP, and some therapeutic effects might have occurred.

A further consideration is that a variation in CPAP compliance existed among Group B participants, which in turn might have influenced the degree of treatment effect. Therefore, we reviewed the CPAP utilization data for Group B participants and defined compliance as the utilization rate per date between PSG and TR.

To evaluate the treatment effect between PSG and TR, we considered the difference between the amount of vitality change before and after sleep at TR (that is, (4)–(3)) and that before and after sleep at PSG (that is, (2)–(1)) to be a measure of such compliance. For the participants in Group B, we calculated CPAP compliance and the relationship between the difference in the amount of vitality change (Fig. 17.5). Although the sample size was limited, at least for participants with less than 90% CPAP utilization on a date-by-date basis, the amount of vitality change in TR did not exceed that in PSG, suggesting that the treatment effect of CPAP could not be achieved. The difference in the amount of vitality change tended to be higher for participants in Group B who maintained a CPAP utilization rate of 90% or higher than those in Group A (significance level $p < 0.1$) and significantly higher for those in Group B with a CPAP utilization rate of less than 90% (significance level $p < 0.05$), as shown in Fig. 17.5. The participants in Group B with low CPAP utilization tended to have a lower difference in the amount of vitality change than those in Group A because the participants in Group B started CPAP before TR owing to the severity of their SAS, and it was desirable to start treatment as early as possible.

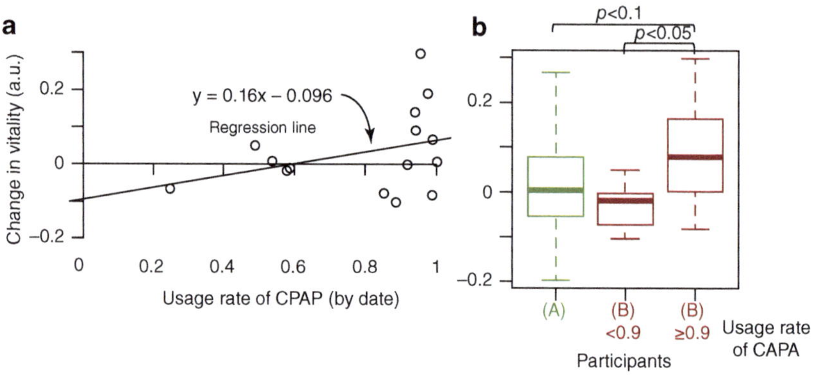

Fig. 17.5 (**a**) Scatterplot for Group B between compliance of CPAP and change in effect of recovery through sleep. Compliance of CPAP is calculated by date: ratio of the number of nights using CPAP to the total number of nights between the first PSG and the titration. The duration of CPAP usage each night is ignored. The effect of recovery through sleep is defined as the subtraction of vitality immediately before sleep from vitality immediately after sleep. (**b**) Boxplot of change in effect of recovery through sleep for each participant group. Group B was classified by the usage rate of CPAP, and its threshold was set at 0.9. (Modified from Nakamura et al. 2018)

Therefore, the severity of their SAS might have been more severe than in Group A. This severity of SAS may affect the distribution shown in Fig. 17.5.

Because MIMOSYS vitality indicates the overall health of an individual and because the algorithm was developed initially to detect major depression, it is difficult to examine the effects of illnesses other than major depression using a simple measurement. However, this study shows that MIMOSYS vitality can be used to estimate the presence or severity of such illnesses if the conditions under which they are likely to have a significant impact are appropriately selected.

17.3 Evaluation of Risk of OSA from Change in Acoustic Features Between Body Position

Next, in addition to the versatile MIMOSYS algorithm, we discuss the development of a voice index specific to SAS.

As the main symptoms of SAS occur during sleep, there are obstacles to measuring the physical condition related to the symptoms by voice. However, it is known that OSA is caused by the physical obstruction of the airway. There are several findings regarding risk factors for OSA; obesity is a risk factor for OSA, and the dimensions of the airway significantly influence the risk of OSA. For example, Japanese people generally have small jawbones and a high prevalence of OSA. In other words, if the airway is narrow, obstruction is likely to occur. AHI is also known to change with body position because the airway shape changes with body position, which, in turn, changes the likelihood of obstruction.

In terms of the mechanism of human speech production, in voiced sounds, the original sound is produced when expiratory air passes through the vocal cords. The specific frequency band components of this sound are emphasized by resonance owing to the structure of the upper airway, and the pattern of these frequency components forms the speech characteristics as a formant. Therefore, if we can determine the resonance from the sound spectrum, we can obtain information regarding the airway shape. However, it is challenging to estimate the dimensions of the airway shape because of its complexity. Therefore, in this study, we asked participants to read the same text in two positions (sitting and supine) and attempted to obtain information on the likelihood of airway obstruction from the speech features affected by differences in position.

The participants in the study were the same as those in the study in which MIMOSYS vitality was calculated from the speech uttered before and after PSG and TR. Its relationship with SAS was investigated, and the voice recorded in the sitting position was analyzed by MIMOSYS. This voice and the voice recorded in the supine position were processed using openSMILE (Eyben et al. 2013) to generate two sets of voice features. The difference or ratio of the corresponding features was adopted as a new feature, and the degree of feature change caused by the difference in body position was evaluated. The correlation between these features and AHI obtained using PSG was investigated.

For example, a scatterplot of the difference in the probability of certainty that the voice is a voiced sound with AHI was plotted (Fig. 17.6a).

The participants were stratified based on symptom severity according to AHI, and the distribution of the speech feature in the scatterplot was plotted (Fig. 17.6b) as a box-and-whisker diagram. Significant differences in this feature were observed, particularly for patients with severe SAS with AHI > 40.

By combining these features appropriately, we expect to predict the likelihood of airway obstruction more precisely and, hence, predict the risk of OSA. In a pilot study, a model combining 33 features was constructed with higher accuracy (Fig. 17.7).

17.4 Conclusions

Sleep-related disorders tend to be more challenging to recognize than other disorders. However, considering the significant impact of sleep disorders on health, technologies to screen sleep disorders in daily life will significantly contribute to achieving healthy longevity. Although it is difficult to acquire voice information during sleep, we have shown that the risk of sleep disorders can be assessed based on voice data obtained during waking hours using ideas such as the timing of voice acquisition, for example, before and after sleep, or by changing the body position.

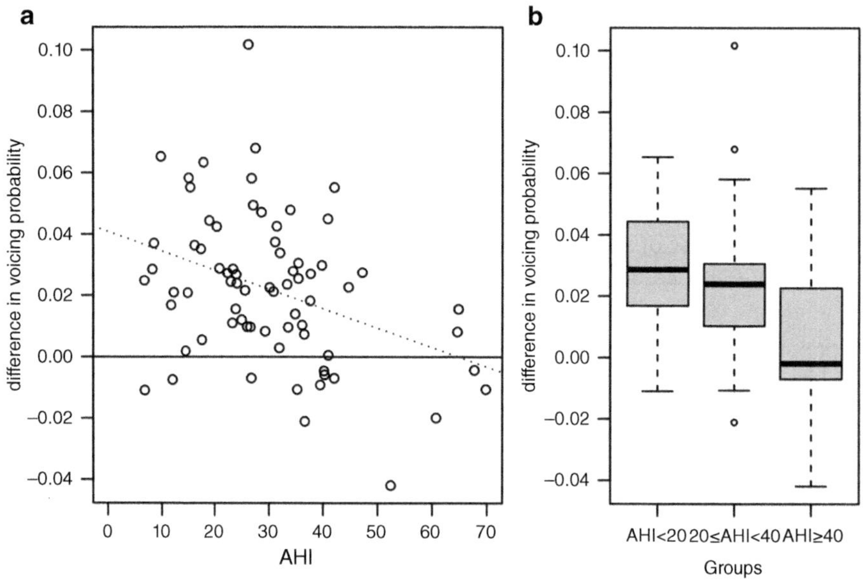

Fig. 17.6 (**a**) Scatterplot between AHI evaluated using PSG and difference in voicing probability by body position. Dotted line shows regression line. The two variables show a slight negative correlation (correlation coefficient is −0.37). (**b**) Boxplot of the same acoustic feature between participant groups classified based on severity of SAS. (Modified from Nakamura et al. 2019)

Fig. 17.7 Pilot model for prediction of AHI from acoustic features measured in two different body positions. Dotted line shows regression line. The correlation coefficient between actual AHI and the predicted index is 0.68. (Modified from Nakamura et al. 2019)

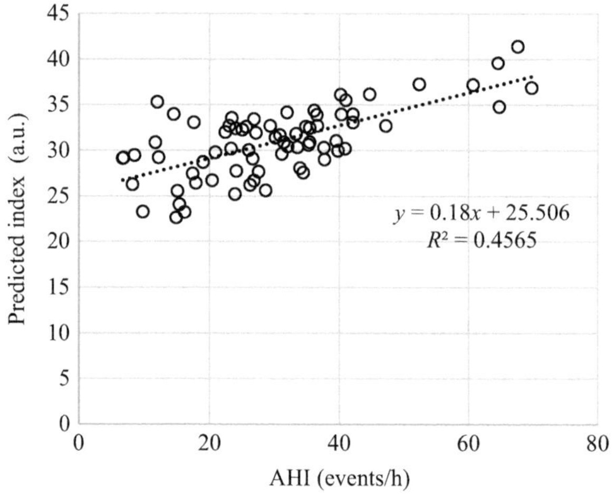

References

Eyben F, Weninger F, Gross F, Schuller B (2013) Recent developments in openSMILE, the Munich open-source multimedia feature extractor. In: Proceedings of the 21st ACM international conference on multimedia, Barcelona, 21–25 October 2013, pp 835–838

Findley LJ, Unverzagt ME, Suratt PM (1998) Automobile accidents involving patients with obstructive sleep apnea. Am Rev Respir Dis 138:337–340
Goldberg DP (1978) Manual of the general health questionnaire. NFER, Windsor
Lavie P, Herer P, Hoffstein V (2000) Obstructive sleep apnoea syndrome as a risk factor for hypertension: population study. BMJ 320:479–482
Mitsuyoshi S, Ren F, Tanaka Y, Kuroiwa S (2006) Non-verbal voice emotion analysis system. Int J Innov Comput 2:819–830
Nakamura M, Shinohara S, Omiya Y, Mitsuyoshi S, Takagi H, Ushiwatari A, Tokuno S (2015) Correlation between self-administered psychological test and emotion measured by voice analysis. In: International conference on information science and management engineering (ICISME2015), Phuket, 20–21 December 2015, pp 290–294.
Nakamura M, Shinohara S, Omiya Y, Mitsuyoshi S, Higuchi M, Hagiwara N, Takano T, Danno H, Tanaka S, Tokuno S (2018) Feasibility study of evaluation of therapeutic effect for sleep apnea syndrome using mental healthiness evaluated from voice. In: IFMBE proceedings 68/2, Praha, 3–8 June 2018, pp 897–900
Nakamura M, Omiya Y, Shinohara S, Higuchi M, Takano T, Mitsuyoshi S, Tanaka S, Tokuno S (2019) Improvement of risk prediction of obstructive sleep apnea syndrome using change in acoustic features dependent on body position [Translated from Japanese] In: Abstract of the 58th annual conference of japanese society for medical and biological engineering, Ginowan, 6–8 June 2019 (in Japanese)
Omiya Y, Hagiwara N, Shinohara S, Nakamura M, Mitsuyoshi S, Tokuno S (2016) Development of mind monitoring system using call voice. In: Abstracts of neuroscience 2016, San Diego, 12–16 November 2016
Ruehland WR, Rochford PD, O'Donoghue FJ, Pierce RJ, Singh P, Thornton AT (2009) The new AASM criteria for scoring hypopneas: impact on the apnea hypopnea index. Sleep 32:150–157
Ryan S, Taylor CT, McNicholas WT (2005) Selective activation of inflammatory pathways by intermittent hypoxia in obstructive sleep apnea syndrome. Circulation 112:2660–2667
Sharafkhaneh A, Giray N, Richardson P, Young T (2005) Association of psychiatric disorders and sleep apnea in a large cohort. Sleep 28:1405–1411
Tasali E, Mokhlesi B, Cauter EV (2008) Obstructive sleep apnea and type 2 diabetes. Chest 133:496–506

Chapter 18
Ankyloglossia with Deviation of the Epiglottis and Larynx (ADEL)

Yasuhiro Omiya

18.1 Introduction

Ankyloglossia with deviation of the epiglottis and larynx (ADEL), in which the origin of the tongue is positioned anteriorly resulting in suppressed breathing, is considered one of the causes of abnormal crying in infants, including night crying and temper tantrums. Moreover, laryngomalacia is another disease that causes inspiratory wheezing in infants. Wheezing is caused by the common cold, respiratory syncytial (RS) virus, asthma, bronchitis, pneumonia, and aspiration. Crying is an important form of expression for infants as it is their way of communicating with their caregivers and others around them. However, the crying of infants suffering from ADEL or laryngomalacia is unpleasant and may be a factor of child abuse, which has become a social problem recently, as parents present have difficulty with childcare, such as temper tantrums.

Simple detection of ADEL and laryngomalacia is an effective way to assist caregivers unfamiliar with childcare in the early detection of the disease and treatment. This chapter presents the development of an algorithm to detect ADEL and laryngomalacia from infant cries.

Y. Omiya (✉)
Research and Development Department, PST Inc., Yokohama, Kanagawa, Japan
e-mail: omiya@medical-pst.com

S. Tokuno, H. Nakamura (eds.), *Voice Biomarkers*,
https://doi.org/10.1007/978-981-96-3109-4_18

18.2 Analysis of Baby's Crying Voice Before and After Correction of the Glosso-Larynx (CGL)

The treatment of ADEL includes correction of the glosso-larynx (CGL) procedure, in which several bundles of the genioglossus muscle are cut from the underside of the tongue. As a result of the procedure, the tongue, epiglottis, and larynx move downward, suppressing breathing due to ADEL and improving breathing due to CGL, as shown in Fig. 18.1.

Thus, CGL improves breathing problems by moving the tongue, glottis, and larynx back and forth, where both the larynx and tongue are erect. It has been reported that symptoms of ADEL and laryngomalacia are improved after corrective laryngectomy (CGL) (Mukai et al. 1991; Mukai and Nitta 2002; Mukai and Yamamoto 2011).

Therefore, the above summarizes an analysis to clarify the differences in the crying sounds of ADEL children before and after CGL treatment which is important to develop basic technologies for the early detection of severe ADEL children to deal with childcare difficulties and take measures such as CGL treatment and childcare support (Omiya et al. 2017).

The crying voices were collected from 106 participants that visited a clinic for CGL surgery. Voices were recorded using a microphone (CO-100K, Sanken) and a portable recorder (R-26, Roland) before and after the CGL procedure. Noiseless crying voices were then extracted using a sound editing software (SoundEngine Free). The crying voices were analyzed using Sensibility Technology (ST) (Mitsuyoshi et al. 2006) and Mind Monitoring System (MIMOSYS) (Shinohara et al. 2021) to extract six features that were then compared and examined before and after CGL.

In ST, five emotion indices (C, A, J, S, and E) were calculated for each utterance, and in MIMOSYS, the vitality index (M) was calculated from the ST results. These six indices were used to detect subtle differences in the timbre of the voice. The present analysis was not conducted from the perspective of emotion or mental health

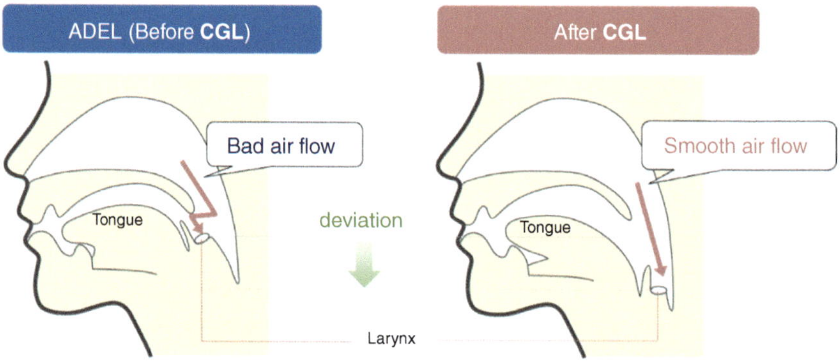

Fig. 18.1 ADEL and CGL

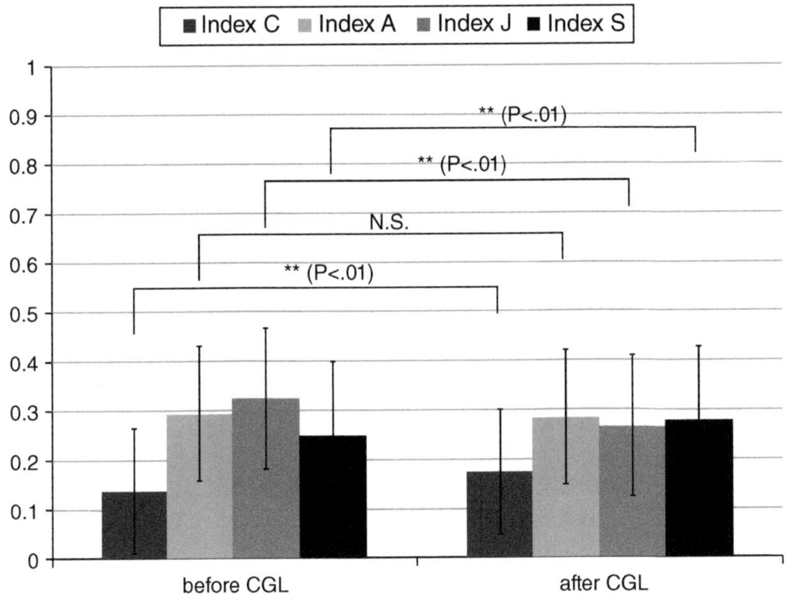

Fig. 18.2 Comparison of indices C, A, J, and S

status, but rather as a scale for measuring changes in the tone quality of voice before and after the CGL treatment. One unit of analysis was defined as one breath of crying.

The distributions of the six features derived using ST and MIMOSYS in the crying voices before and after the CGL treatment are shown in Figs. 18.2 and 18.3. The mean of each indice was verified by a t-test, where significant differences were found for five indices (indice C: $t(1921) = -6.448, p < 0.01$; indice J: $t(1921) = 8.136, p < 0.01$; indice S: $t(1921) = -4.429, p < 0.01$; indice E: $t(1921) = 7.046, p < 0.01$; index M: $t(1921) = 3.447, p < 0.01$). These results suggest that the downward movement of the tongue, epiglottis, and larynx changes the tone quality of the crying voice.

18.3 Identification of Laryngomalacia by Baby's Crying Voice

Laryngomalacia is the most common cause of inspiratory wheezing in infants, and wheezing is often seen in crying and is commonly caused by the common cold, RS virus, asthma, bronchitis, pneumonia, and aspiration. The simple detection of laryngomalacia is effective for its early detection and treatment. Therefore, we investigated an algorithm to detect laryngomalacia from infant crying sounds (Omiya et al. 2019).

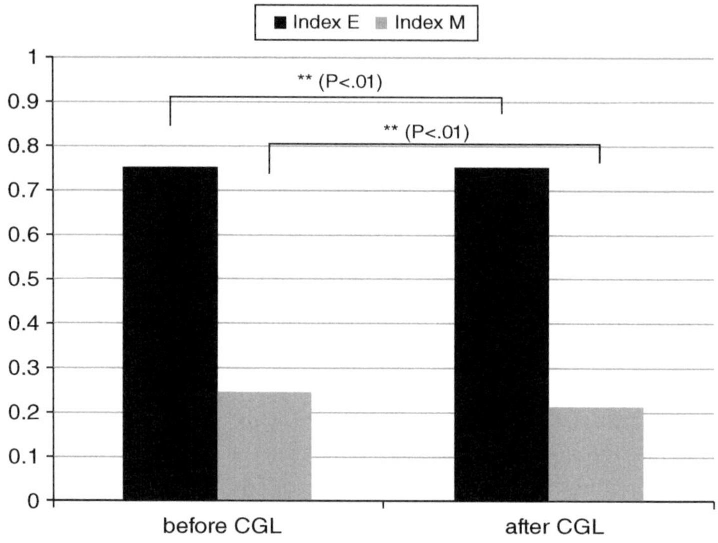

Fig. 18.3 Comparison before and after CGL indices E and M

Table 18.1 Classification matrix

		Classified	
		Laryngomalacia	Not laryngomalacia
Actual	Laryngomalacia	79	15
	Not laryngomalacia	11	55

Infant participants that visited a clinic for the CGL surgery were recorded using a microphone (CO-100K, Sanken) and a portable recorder (R-26, Roland) before and after the CGL procedure, and a physician diagnosed the presence or absence of laryngomalacia. Of 101 participants, 64 were diagnosed with laryngomalacia. Next, noise-free crying voices were extracted from the recorded audio files using a sound editing software (SoundEngine Free). The extracted cries ranged from 1 to 89 depending on the participant.

In the analysis, 6552 acoustic features were analyzed from chirping speech using openSMILE version 2.3 (Eyben et al. 2010). Next, an algorithm was created to distinguish laryngomalacia using the LightGBM Python package (Ke et al. 2017) through the holdout method with 20% as test data. For the training data, 359 speech data diagnosed as laryngomalacia and 277 speech data diagnosed as normal were used. For the validation data, 94 speech data diagnosed as laryngomalacia and 66 speech data diagnosed as normal were used.

As shown in Table 18.1, the classification performance of the algorithm for discerning laryngomalacia from the crying voice was 84.0%, 83.3%, and 83.8%, sensitivity, specificity, and accuracy, respectively. These results suggest that it may be possible to capture the speech characteristics of laryngomalacia using crying sounds.

18.4 Summary

The development of an algorithm was described for detecting ADEL and laryngomalacia from infant cries, and differences in the speech indices derived from the cries before and after CGL treatment were found, suggesting that tongue and larynx deviation changes the cries. In addition, a discrimination algorithm for the presence or absence of laryngomalacia was developed, and the correct response rate in the validation data exceeded 80%, suggesting that the voice characteristics of laryngomalacia can be captured by the crying sounds. These results suggest that the analysis of crying voices of infants who are not breathing normally may lead to the detection of ADEL and laryngomalacia and that appropriate treatment may contribute to the improvement of symptoms of inappropriate childcare and avoidance of sudden infant death syndrome.

References

Eyben F, Wöllmer M, Schuller B (2010) openSMILE—the Munich versatile and fast open-source audio feature extractor. In: Proceedings of the 18th ACM international conference on Multimedia, Firenze, pp 1459–1462

Ke G, Meng Q, Finley T, Wang T, Chen W, Ma W, Ye Q, Liu TY (2017) LightGBM: a highly efficient gradient boosting decision tree. Adv Neural Inf Proces Syst 30(NIPS 2017):3146–3154

Mitsuyoshi S, Ren F, Tanaka Y, Kuroiwa S (2006) Non-verbal voice emotion analysis system. Int J ICIC 2:819–830

Mukai S, Nitta M (2002) Correction of the glossolarynx (CGL) and resultant positional changes of the hyoid bone and cranium. Acta Otolaryngol Sweden September 2002(122):644–650

Mukai S, Yamamoto I (2011) Partial genioglossectomy leading to an increase in respiratory rate—surgery for ankyloglossia with deviation of the epiglottis and larynx. Ann ADEL 16:25–31

Mukai S, Mukai C, Asaoka K (1991) Congenital ankyloglossia with deviation of the epiglottis and larynx. Ann Otolaryngol 100:1–20

Omiya Y, Yamamoto I, Nakamura M, Shinohara S, Mitsuyoshi S, Tokuno S, Nakagawa K, Fukuchi Y, Mukai S (2017) Analysis of baby's crying voice before and after CGL—follow-up report—[Translated from Japanese]. Ann ADEL 21:70–71. (in Japanese)

Omiya Y, Nakamura S, Shinohara S, Higuchi M, Suzuki K, Manome N, Mitsuyoshi S, Yamamoto I, Mukai S, Tokuno S (2019) An experiment to detect Laryngomalacia using baby's crying voice. In: The 41st international engineering in medicine and biology conference (EMBC 2019), Berlin, 23–27 July 2019

Shinohara S, Nakamura M, Omiya Y, Higuchi M, Hagiwara N, Mitsuyoshi S, Toda H, Saito T, Tanichi M, Yoshino A, Tokuno S (2021) Depressive mood assessment method based on emotion level derived from voice: comparison of voice features of individuals with major depressive disorders and healthy controls. Int J Environ Res Public Health 18(10):5435

Chapter 19
Ultrasonic Vocalization (USV)

Mitsuteru Nakamura

19.1 Introduction

The main objective of our research group was to understand mental and physical conditions and diseases in humans by analyzing the indirect effects of these diseases on human speech.

Although human speech, as a means of communication, is significantly more developed than that of other animals, there are animals other than humans that communicate through vocalization. For example, bird songs have been studied intensively as a learning model for language (Wilbrecht and Nottebohm 2003). In utilizing language as a means of communication, it is necessary to communicate symbolic content such that the acoustic signals are not distinguished deliberately from similar ones within a same linguistic element. Many animal vocalization researchers interpret acoustic signals according to the context.

However, animal vocalization, like human speech, as noted above, can be characterized by unintended signal changes owing to disease. Although the characteristics of vocal mechanisms and vocalization signals of animals and humans vary significantly and findings in humans are not directly applicable to animals, it is possible to apply speech analysis techniques to animal vocalization by appropriately modifying the frequency range and other parameters.

The practical significance of research on animal voice is its ability to reveal the health status of pets, livestock, and other animals, similar to research on human speech. In the field of medicine, voice analysis technique enables noninvasive evaluation of the efficacy of new drug candidates, the toxicity of chemical substances, and effect of genome editing. This noninvasiveness reduces the number of required

M. Nakamura (✉)
Department of Bioengineering, Graduate School of Engineering, The University of Tokyo, Bunkyo-ku, Tokyo, Japan
e-mail: nakamura@bioeng.t.u-tokyo.ac.jp

S. Tokuno, H. Nakamura (eds.), *Voice Biomarkers*,
https://doi.org/10.1007/978-981-96-3109-4_19

animal subjects and consequently contribute to ethical use of animals and reduction of research costs.

Rodents, such as mice and rats, are some of the most widely used animals in medical research aimed at making findings that are transferable to humans. As mammals, these animals have some similarities with humans. Furthermore, their rapid growth and small size make research periods short and costs relatively low. The establishment of specific strains and knockout/knock-in techniques for mice makes it easy to clarify the relationship among diseases, physical characteristics, and genes.

Although rodents such as mice and rats emit sounds that are audible to humans, they generally conduct intraspecies communication through ultrasonic vocalization (USV). This vocalization is achieved in the ultrasonic band whose frequency is above the human audible range.

Both rodents are known to produce USV in different frequency ranges depending on the context. For instance, the USV produced by males during intragender territorial disputes varies from the one they emit when they are courting the females, which is also distinct from the one produced by pups separated from their mothers (Portfors 2007).

As mentioned above, the USVs emitted by mice separated from their mothers is generally classified into approximately ten types (Scattoni et al. 2008) based on the patterns of change in both the time and frequency axes of the vocalization signals observed on the spectrogram. However, it is unclear whether this pattern classification has valid implications for auditory information processing in mice.

In addition, the vocalization produced by the pups is an acoustic cue for the mother to search for them. This is even more important in the case of pups that are approximately 1-week old, owing to their limited mobility, which makes it difficult for them to move to their mothers.

19.2 Prediction of Social Behaviors Related to Autism Spectrum Disorders Using Analysis of Call-Type Patterns of USVs Elicited in Pups by Maternal Separation

19.2.1 Introduction

We created a mouse model of autism spectrum disorder (ASD) in humans, focusing on copy number variants (Matsumoto et al. 2017; Hiroi and Nishi 2015; Hiroi and Yamauchi 2019). We studied pups separated from their mothers and analyzed their vocalization. Epidemiological studies have shown that ASD is a communication disorder with significant genetic components (Abrahams and Geschwind 2008). Subsequently, we have described the study, wherein pups were separated from their dams at 8 (PND8) and 12 (PND12) days old. The subjects were mice in which the gene corresponding to the human 16p11.2 gene, a known risk factor for ASD in humans (Niarchou et al. 2019), had been knocked out and wild-type mice as a control group. The USVs emitted by the pups were recorded over a 5-min period during the maternal separation. The phenotype of social behavior was examined at 1 month old using a test battery for assessing social behavior, and the predictability of social behavior postmaturity based on the characteristics of the USVs in the neonatal period was examined.

19.2.2 Methods

In analyzing the USV of mice and rats, the unit of analysis is a vocalization signal called a call, a continuous acoustic power over time. A call corresponds to the utterance unit in human speech analysis. In this study, calls were manually detected and categorized using assist by software, and time-series data on call types were obtained. To determine whether two consecutive calls constituted a continuous sequence or not, the frequency distribution was examined by varying the threshold of the call interval length, which was considered to be a nonconsecutive break in the sequence. The value at which the distribution changed significantly was considered to be the maximum call interval at which the sequence was continuous. The USVs emitted by pups separated from their mother were classified into 12 types, based on the proposed typology. The order of their appearance was analyzed using the Markov model. In this study, the call types were abbreviated as follows: complex (Cx), two syllables (Ts), frequency steps (Fs), harmonics (Ha), composite (C), hump (H), short (Sh), downward (D), flat (F), upward (U), ambiguous (Am), and uncharacterized (Un). The pups that produced less than ten calls in a 5-min recording were excluded from the analysis as it may not be possible to properly evaluate the proportion of the call types.

On the other hand, a test battery was used to assess postmaturity social behavior in the following order: the reciprocal social interactions, approach to novel objects, olfactory responses to various odorants, spontaneous alternation in the T-maze, the elevated plus maze, locomotor activity and thigmotaxis in an inescapable open field, startle response, and prepulse inhibition. The genotype of the knockout mice was also confirmed using RNA-seq.

19.2.3 Results

In the figures given below, the test group, the knockout mice, is denoted as Del/+, indicating that the target gene was knocked out heterozygously, and the control group, the wild type, is denoted as +/+. As shown in Fig. 19.1a, based on the genotypes, there was no statistically significant difference in terms of the frequency of each type of call and the number of vocalizations of all the USVs. In the

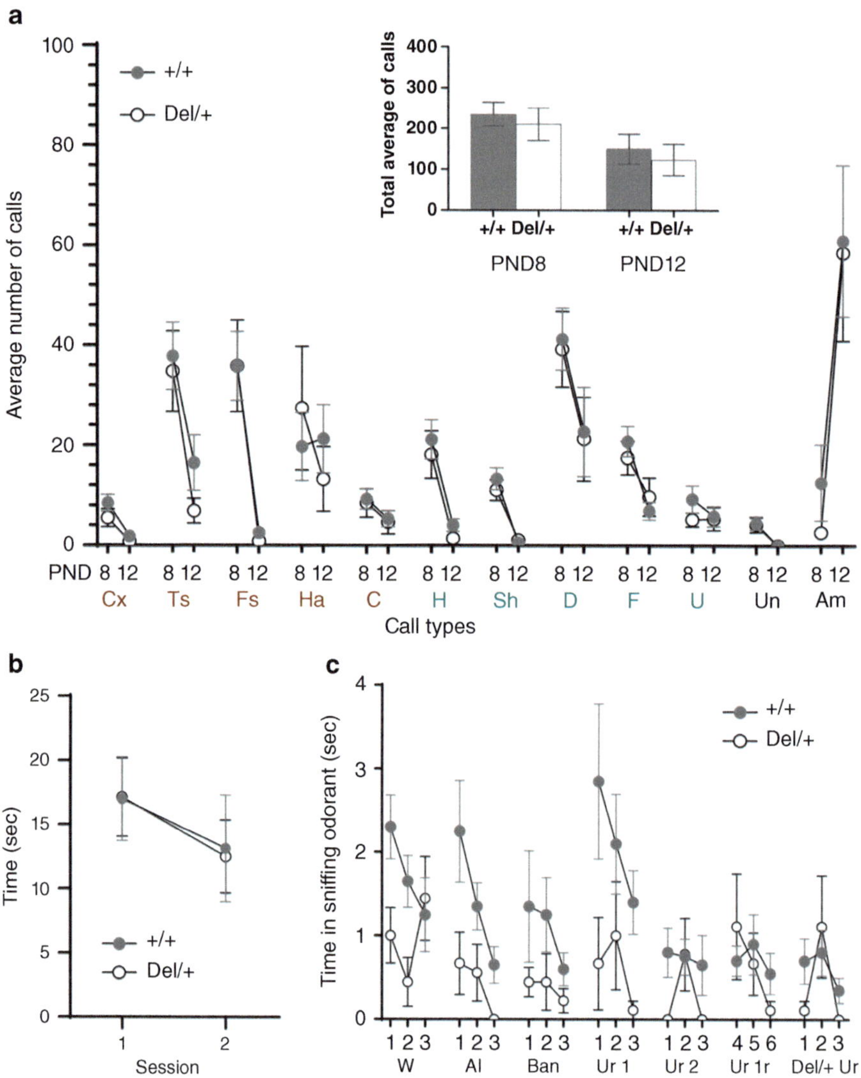

Fig. 19.1 (**a**) Number of calls emitted by both groups of mice. Number of each call type is shown in the main panel, and the total number of calls through call types are shown in inset. Call types are abbreviated. (**b**) Social interaction. Social interaction was measured twice, sequentially (Sessions 1 and 2). (**c**) Olfactory responses. Responses were measured three times sequentially for each olfactory stimulus. Types of olfactory stimuli are abbreviated. *W* water, *Al* almond, *Ban* banana, *Ur 1* urine of other wild type; Mouse 1, *Ur 2* urine of other wild type; Mouse 2 (different from Mouse 1), *Del/+ Ur* urine of mouse with knocked-out gene. Ur 1 was examined twice, just before Ur 2 and just after Ur 2. (Modified from Nakamura et al. 2021)

postmaturity behavioral test, as shown in Fig. 19.1b, based on the genotypes, there were no significant differences in the social interaction, which is the approach toward other individuals. In terms of the responses to odor stimuli, no statistically significant differences were observed, except for the olfactory response to urine of an unfamiliar wild-type mouse, as shown in Fig. 19.1c. To measure the responses to olfactory stimuli, three successive measurement sessions were conducted. Linear model analysis confirmed that the responses decreased as sessions were repeated, i.e., novelty was lost. In this study, the difference or amount of change in the olfactory response between the first and third sessions was attributed to the habituation of the olfactory response and was the subject of subsequent analyses. In addition, because only a few individuals at PND 12 emitted USVs at a frequency that could be analyzed, subsequent analyses will focus on the USVs emitted by the mice at PND 8.

We then proceeded to investigate the possibility of obtaining useful indices for predicting social behaviors by analyzing the USVs. The target behaviors to be predicted were olfactory responses to odor stimuli that indicated significant differences based on genotypes and social interaction. The olfactory response was calculated as the percentage of total time spent approaching odorants during the 2-min measurement period, and the social interaction was determined based on the time spent in approaching other individuals. We analyzed the relationship between the number of Markov model transitions referring to the previous call type and the entropy of the sequence when the sequence of the call types was interpreted using the Markov model. Because the most significant difference between the genotypes was observed in the 2-gram case, only the association between two consecutive call types was considered, such that the transition of a call type was affected only by the preceding call type.

Three approaches were used in this study to extract patterns for behavior prediction from the two consecutive call-type transition patterns analyzed. The first approach was to investigate the relationship between the individual features selected by the regression algorithm to build models and indices for predicting social behaviors. In the models, the probability and frequency of call-type transitions, the probability and frequency of occurrence of call types without history, and some acoustic features calculated using the USV recording software (Avisoft-SASLab Pro, Avisoft Bioacoustics, Glienicke/Nordbahn, Germany) to assist in USV detection were used as candidate explanatory variables. The models were derived using LASSO linear regression (Tibshirani 1996) to predict one of the four quantitative indices for social behaviors as the target variable. Second, using the same set of candidate explanatory variables as was used for the first model, a predictive model was derived using the LASSO logistic regression based on the genotype difference between the knockout mice and wild-type mice as the objective variable; then, the relationship between the social behaviors and features expected to show the differences between the genotypes selected by the algorithm were examined. Third, we examined the relationship between social behaviors and transitions between two consecutive call types in the Markov model, whose probability was statistically significantly higher than that

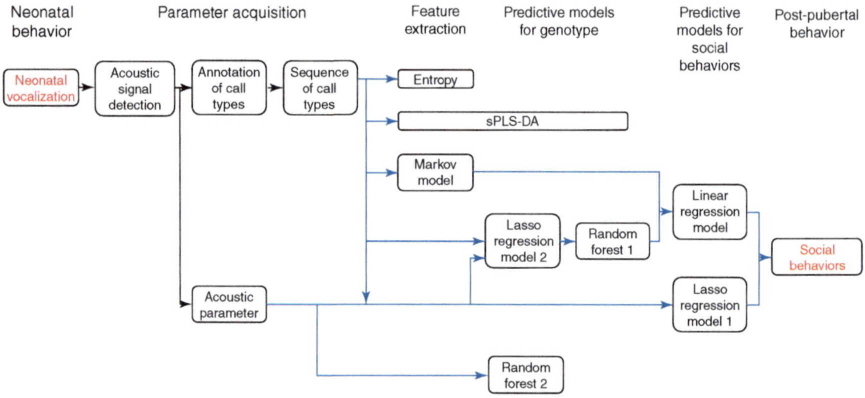

Fig. 19.2 Diagram of analysis. There are three paths for social behavior prediction: LASSO regression model 1 for direct behavior prediction, linear regression after LASSO regression model 2 for genotype prediction, and linear regression after the Markov model. Black arrows show preparation process for acquiring the parameters, i.e., explanatory variables in the prediction models, and blue arrows show the modelling process using the acquired parameters. (Modified from Nakamura et al. 2021)

of transitions in the model in which the call type appeared when history was not considered. The flow of these analyses is shown in Fig. 19.2.

As the first of the three approaches mentioned above, we present the results of LASSO regression model 1, which constructed a regression model to predict post-maturity social behavior using variables related to call type and other acoustic features as the explanatory variables. Figure 19.3 shows the relationship between the fraction deviance explained in the prediction model and the coefficients of the explanatory variables used in the model. Figure 19.3a–d indicates the coefficient values of the explanatory variables in the models, predicting social interaction, social interaction habituation, olfactory response, and olfactory response habituation, respectively. The variables with strong explanatory power, which were selected when one-fourth of all the deviations were explained by the linear regression model, to avoid overfitting, are labeled in the figure. These labels indicate that most of them were related to the type transition between two consecutive calls. Furthermore, majority of the variables with weak explanatory power were related to type transitions between the two calls, as well (not shown in Fig. 19.3).

Thereafter, we examined the logistic LASSO regression model 2 that predicts the genotype itself based on the same set of the USV-related variables as before, instead of indices related to postmaturity social behavior. In this case, as shown in Fig. 19.4, we confirmed that many variables related to the type of transition between the two calls were selected. To examine the explanatory ability of the variables selected in this model, a classifier that predicted the genotype from the variables selected when the fraction deviance explained was 0.5 was constructed using the random forest method. When a sample obtained from a knockout mouse was defined as positive, the sensitivity and specificity were 0.500 and 0.792, respectively.

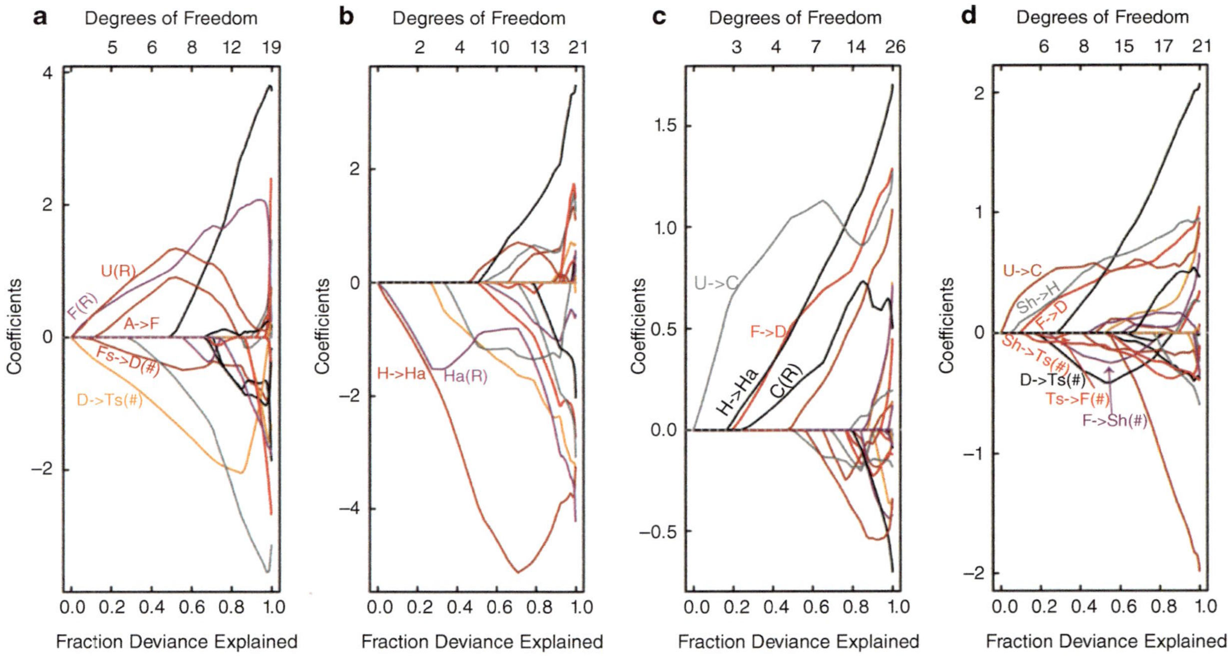

Fig. 19.3 Coefficients of explanatory variables in models to obtain indices for social behavior prediction. The models were acquired through LASSO regression. The horizontal and vertical axes show the fraction deviance, as explained by the model, and the coefficients of parameters, respectively. All parameters (call-type number and ratios, call sequence number and probabilities, acoustic parameters) were used for selection. The objective variable in each model was as follows: (**a**) social interaction; (**b**) social habituation; (**c**) olfactory response; (**d**) olfactory habituation. Habituations in social interaction and olfactory response were defined as the difference between the scores at the first and last trials, i.e., Trial 2 score—Trial 1 score for social interaction and Trial 3 score—Trial 1 score for the olfactory response. The labeled traces show the explanatory variables with nonzero coefficient at 0.25 of the fraction deviance explained. The variables related to two-call sequence are labelled "X->Y," where X and Y indicate the types of preceding and succeeding calls, respectively, i.e., a two-call sequence, wherein F is the first call and Sh is the second call, is labelled as "F->Sh." The labels for the number of two-call sequences have a postfix "(#)," unlike those for the probabilities of two-call sequences. The labels for the ratio of the number of a call type emitted to all the calls have a postfix "(R)." The same labelling rule is applied throughout this chapter. (Modified from Nakamura et al. 2021)

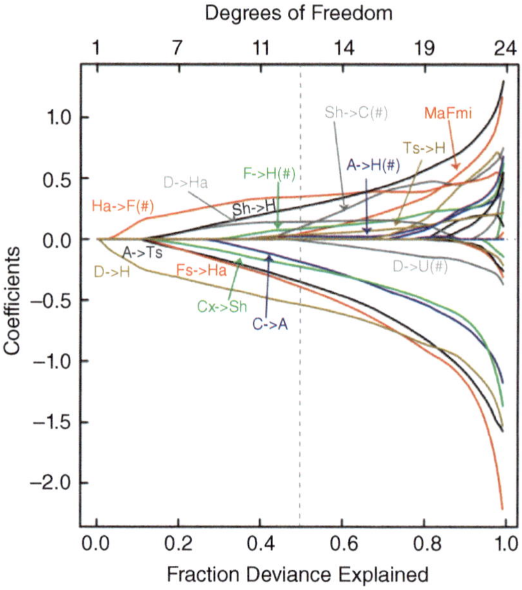

Fig. 19.4 Coefficients of explanatory variables in genotype-predicting models. The models were acquired through LASSO regression. The horizontal and vertical axes show the fraction deviance explained by the model and the coefficients of parameters, respectively. All the parameters (call-type number and ratios, call sequence number and probabilities, acoustic parameters) were used for selection. (Modified from Nakamura et al. 2021)

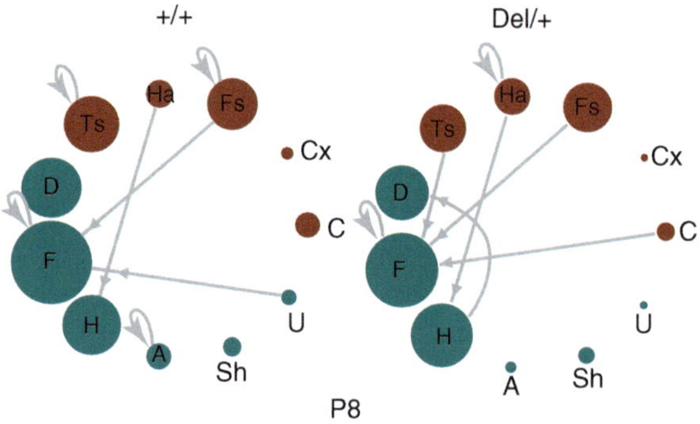

Fig. 19.5 Markov models identified the most frequent call connections between two calls at P8. The labels of each circle indicate the call type, and the arrows between the circles show the most frequently observed two-call sequence. (Modified from Nakamura et al. 2021)

For the third approach, the two-call sequences were determined to have a significantly higher probability of occurrence as sequences in the Markov model than the probability that a call would occur according to the probability of occurrence of a single call type without a history, as shown in Fig. 19.5.

The variables selected based on the three approaches above and those with significant correlations with the indices of social behaviors for each group of genotypes are shown in Fig. 19.6. These results show that, when analyzed based on genotype, many variables involved in the USV call-type transitions were significantly correlated with the indices of social behavior among the wild-type mice. However, such variables were fewer in the knockout mice. In addition, although the random forest classifier, which predicted genotypes based on the variables selected

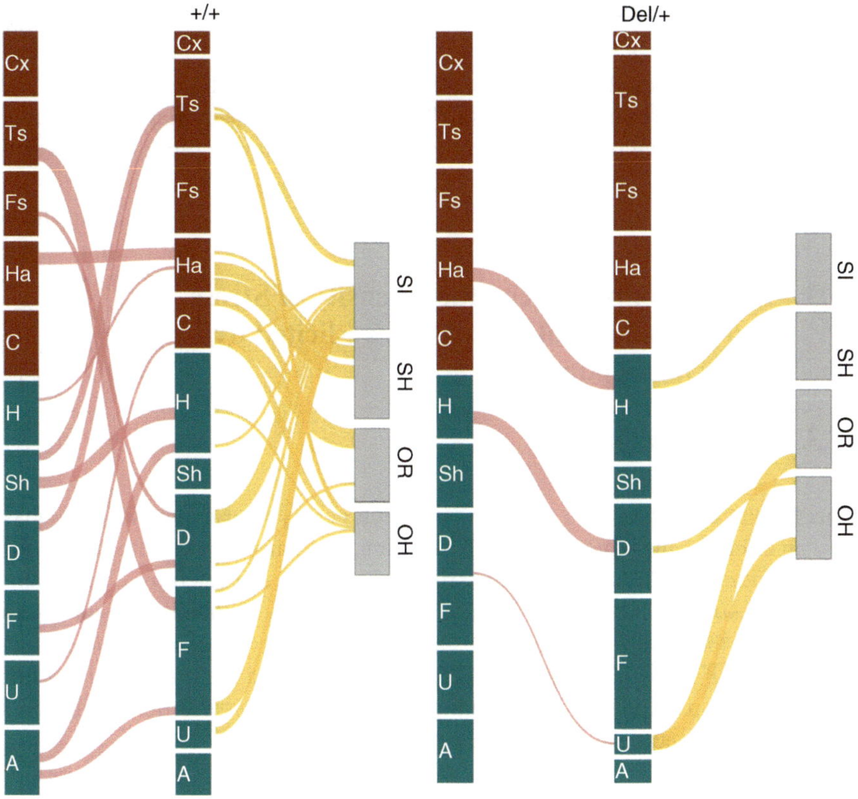

Fig. 19.6 Visualization of the relationships among call types, their sequences, and postpubertal social behaviors. The thickness of each path from one call type to the next represents the proportion of such transition probabilities from one call to another (see pink lines). Only significant correlation coefficients ($p < 0.05$) are shown. The strength of paths predicting each postpubertal social behavior is indicated by the thickness of the lines from the second call column to the postpubertal social behavior column. Only cases in which the goodness of fit was significant are shown (see yellow lines). The thickness of lines with different levels of significance ($p < 0.05$, $p < 0.01$, and $p < 0.001$) are represented by arbitrary thickness units x, 2x, and 4x, respectively. The postpubertal social behavior indices are abbreviated as follows: SI, social interaction; SH, habituation of social interaction; OR, olfactory response; OH, habituation of olfactory response. (Modified from Nakamura et al. 2021)

using the second approach, had a high specificity for correctly determining the wild type, it had a low sensitivity for correctly determining the knockout. This suggested that the association between the USV-type transition pattern and social behavior was weaker in the knockout mice, possibly leading to greater atypicality in the vocal behavior.

19.2.4 Conclusion

Thus, it can be concluded that the relationship between multiple calls in the call type-based analysis of neonatal mouse USVs may predict the social behavior after maturation, indicating that USVs in early development may facilitate early diagnosis of ASD.

19.3 Relationship Between the Intensity of Stress and Acoustic Features of USVs Elicited by Maternal Separation

19.3.1 Introduction

Thus far, we have described situations in which genotype or expression type may have an effect on the pattern of call. Apart from the changes in voice owing to the presence of certain diseases or disease risk factors, pups separated from their dams experience stress. The features of the USV emitted by isolated pups may vary according to the intensity of the stress. One example of a condition that could affect the intensity of stress is the distance between the pups and their dams. To test this possibility, we recorded the USVs emitted by isolated pups at different distances from their dams and analyzed their acoustic features.

19.3.2 Methods

We used wild-type rats as the subjects in this study. The measurements were made at the several distances using the same dam-pup pairs. Owing to the sequential changes in the distance between the rearing cages, changes might be observed over time. By sequentially increasing the distance between the cages in the first half of the measurement and decreasing the distance between the cages in reverse order in the second half, we confirmed that the change in the feature of the USVs solely depended on the distance, not on the time. The positions of the cages where the USVs were recorded and the order in which they were recorded are shown in Fig. 19.7. In each measurement condition, recordings were made for 5 min, and maximum efforts were made to keep the interval between the measurement conditions as short as possible.

We examined the effects of conditions of rats on the acoustic features under four conditions: 1-week and 2-week-old rats, with and without a heating pad. Although the frequency of the rat USV is significantly higher than that of human speech, the acoustic features were analyzed using the Sensibility Technology software that was originally designed to extract features from human voice. To obtain meaningful results, the sampling frequency of the recorded USV was scaled for the analysis.

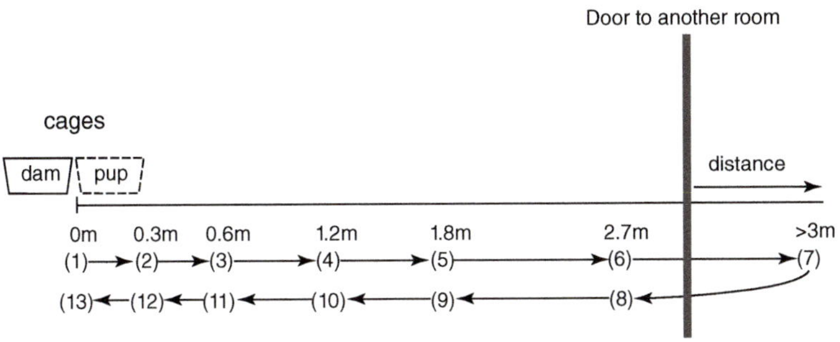

Fig. 19.7 Schematic diagram of measurement conditions. Position of the cage enclosing a dam was fixed, and the cage enclosing a pup was placed at the distance shown in the figure. The distance increased in the first half of the measurement and decreased in the latter half of the measurement. Actual distance between the dam and pup was larger than the distance between the cages, as they could move freely inside the cages

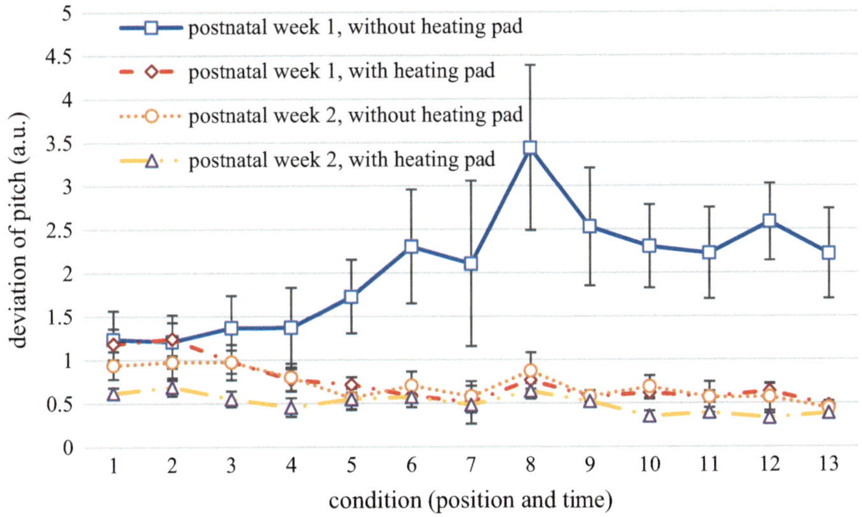

Fig. 19.8 Plot of a specific acoustic feature (deviation of pitch) in each group and measurement conditions. Numbers in horizontal axis correspond to numbers in Fig. 19.7

Therefore, although the calculated values retained the properties of a proportional scale, they did not directly represent the physical quantities.

19.3.3 Results

As shown in Fig. 19.8, the deviation of pitch, an acoustic feature of the USV emitted by 1-week-old pups separated from their dams without a heating pad, reflected distance-dependent changes. However, no such change was observed under the same positional conditions when the pups had heating pads. In addition, no distant-dependent changes were observed in the same acoustic feature of 2-week-old pups, whether they had heating pads or not. This indicated that distance-dependent changes in the acoustic feature were dependent on the age and thermal environment, and the stress experienced by approximately 1-week-old pups was directly proportional to the distance from their dams. However, we did not measure the body temperature of the pups. In the future, we will quantitatively examine the stress experienced by neonatal rats during maternal separation in relation to the changes in the pups' body temperature.

References

Abrahams B, Geschwind D (2008) Advances in autism genetics: on the threshold of a new neurobiology. Nat Rev Genet 9:341–355

Hiroi N, Nishi A (2015) Dimensional deconstruction and reconstruction of CNV-associated neuropsychiatric disorders. In: Pletnikov MV, Waddington JL (eds) Modeling the psychopathological dimensions of schizophrenia: from molecules to behavior, vol 23. London, Elsevier, pp 285–302

Hiroi N, Yamauchi T (2019) Modeling and predicting developmental trajectories of neuropsychiatric dimensions associated with copy number variations. Int J Neuropsychopharmacol 22:488–500

Matsumoto M, Walton NM, Yamada H, Kondo Y, Marek GJ, Tajinda K (2017) The impact of genetics on future drug discovery in schizophrenia. Expert Opin Drug Discov 12:673–686

Nakamura M, Ye K, Barbachan e Silva M, Yamauchi T, Hoeppner DJ, Fayyazuddin A, Kang G, Yuda EA, Nagashima M, Enomoto S, Hiramoto T, Sharp R, Kaneko I, Tajinda K, Adachi M, Mihara T, Tokuno S, Geyer MA, Ó Broin P, Matsumoto M, Hiroi N (2021) Computational identification of variables in neonatal vocalizations predictive for postpubertal social behaviors in a mouse model of 16p11.2 deletion. Mol Psychiatry 26:6578–6588

Niarchou M, Chawner S, Doherty JL, Maillard AM, Jacquemont S, Chung WK, Green-Snyder LA, Bernier RA, Goin-Kochel RP, Hanson E, Linden DEJ, Linden SC, Raymond FL, Skuse D, Hall J, Owen MJ, van den Bree MBM (2019) Psychiatric disorders in children with 16p11.2 deletion and duplication. Transl Psychiatry 9:8

Portfors CV (2007) Types and functions of ultrasonic vocalizations in laboratory rats and mice. J Am Assoc Lab Anim Sci 46:28–34

Scattoni ML, Gandhy SU, Ricceri L, Crawley JN (2008) Unusual repertoire of vocalizations in the BTBR T+tf/J mouse model of autism. PLoS ONE 3:e3067

Tibshirani R (1996) Regression shrinkage and selection via the lasso. J R Stat Soc Ser B Methodol 58(1):267–288

Wilbrecht L, Nottebohm F (2003) Vocal learning in birds and humans. Ment Retard Dev Disabil Res Rev 9:135–148

Chapter 20
Driving

Takeshi Takano

20.1 Introduction

Recent automobiles are equipped with advanced safety technologies and sophisticated information processing systems for various purposes, such as advanced safety technology and information display to the driver. Driver monitoring has attracted considerable attention as an application of these components. There are two major applications for driver monitoring. One is in the field of "infotainment," which improves usability by understanding the driver's context and presenting the appropriate information. The other is in the field of advanced safety technology, which understands whether the driver is ready to drive and provides appropriate intervention.

In this research, technologies for detecting the human mental state from speech were developed, and it is expected that these technologies can be implemented in vehicles. In this chapter, research on detecting the change of mental state of the driver using voice and estimating the driving ability of an elderly driver using voice is introduced.

T. Takano (✉)
Department of Pharmacology, School of Medicine, UT Health San Antonio, San Antonio, TX, USA
e-mail: takanot@uthscsa.edu

S. Tokuno, H. Nakamura (eds.), *Voice Biomarkers*,
https://doi.org/10.1007/978-981-96-3109-4_20

20.2 Detecting the Change of Mental State of the Driver Using Voice

When driving a car, the driver's mental and physical states affect the overall driving operation. Fatigue and drowsiness caused by various diseases, mental health problems, and stress from driving interfere with the accuracy of the recognition, judgment, and operation processes of driving. These factors can increase the risk of severe automobile accidents. To avoid such risks and to create a safe state, a system that monitors the condition of the driver and provides appropriate support is required.

Many methods for estimating the state of the driver have been studied. When limited to experimental driving, direct biological signal measurements, such as electroencephalography and electrocardiography, can be used. However, these methods require complicated equipment to be attached to the driver and are impractical. Compared with these methods, voice analysis is not only noninvasive and noncontact but also does not require special equipment, and it is inexpensive and remote. Therefore, the possibility of using MIMOSYS to detect drivers' mental states was investigated (Okazaki 2016).

In this study, 271 subject drivers were divided into 3 groups and asked to drive 3 vehicles with different characteristics on city roads and highways for approximately 30 min, driving normally with traffic flow. The MIMOSYS and temporary mood scale (TMS; Tokuda 2011) were introduced for evaluating moods of the subjects, and they were conducted before and after the test drives. The experimental procedure is shown in Table 20.1.

Figure 20.1 shows that cars A and B increase the driver's vitality. Figure 20.2 shows the result of change after driving Car A. This indicates that MIMOSYS can detect a driver's positive moods.

Table 20.1 Flow of the experiment

Group A	Group B	Group C
TMS Voice recording	TMS Voice recording	TMS Voice recording
Driving: Car A	Driving: Car B	Driving: Car C
TMS Voice recording	TMS Voice recording	TMS Voice recording
Driving: Car C	Driving: Car A	Driving: Car B
TMS Voice recording	TMS Voice recording	TMS Voice recording
Driving: Car B	Driving: Car C	Driving: Car A
TMS Voice recording	TMS Voice recording	TMS Voice recording

Both the city and the highway test have the same rotating schedule
Adapted and modified from Okazaki (2016)

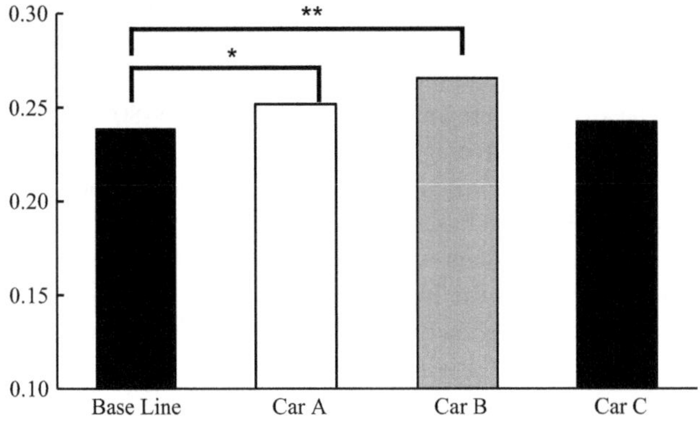

Fig. 20.1 Vitality changes before and after driving on the city course. The baseline means vitality before driving, and the bar for each car shows vitality after driving. Vehicle A: easy to drive car. Vehicle B: sporty car. Vehicle C: comfortable car. (Adapted and modified from Okazaki 2016) Significance level: $*p < 0.05$, $**p < 0.01$

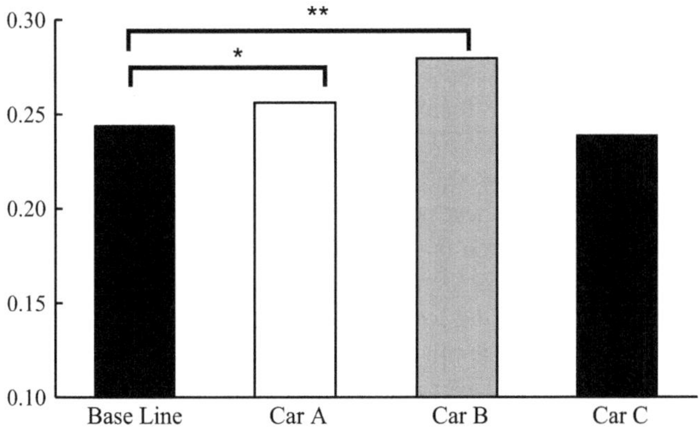

Fig. 20.2 Vitality changes before and after driving on the highway course. (Adapted and modified from Okazaki 2016.) This figure illustrates the same tendency as the city course (Fig. 20.1)

20.3 Estimating the Driving Ability of Elderly Driver Using Voice

The ratio of fatal accidents involving elderly drivers is increasing annually and is of great interest to society. The Japan Geriatrics Society and others have suggested that whether an elderly driver is unfit to drive should not be based on a medical "diagnosis of dementia" but on actual skills judged by experts through driving tests. The judgment of impaired driving ability requires a high level of expertise, time, and cost. The relationship between voice and cognitive function and driving ability in elderly drivers was investigated to provide a simple screening method for the decline of driving ability.

Elderly drivers qualified to drive were recruited, their driving ability was tested using a driving simulator, their cognitive ability was tested using the Mini-Mental State Examination (MMSE), and their speech was collected through the reading of fixed phrases. The drivers were male, N = 24, aged 65–80 (average 70.0), and female, N = 20, aged 65–73 (average 67.8). The driving simulator was an ACCESS CHECKER ACM200 manufactured by Hitachi KE Systems, and the driving skills of the subjects were calculated based on their operations.

The analysis in this experiment was conducted using two approaches. One was a deductive approach based on the hypothesis that drivers with poor driving scores react poorly and speak more slowly. The other was an inductive approach to find features representative of the driving score of the driver among various acoustic parameters.

Figure 20.3 shows a scatterplot of the MMSE and driving scores of the participants in this experiment. The correlation coefficient is 0.03, indicating no correlation between the two. It is difficult to estimate driving skills using the MMSE.

Figure 20.4 shows a scatterplot of the driving score and speed of speech. There is a dominant correlation coefficient of 0.324, suggesting the possibility of estimating driving skills based on speech speed.

Figure 20.5 shows the distribution of the driving ability evaluation index for the high- and low-driving-skill groups. This index was created from 12 useful features extracted from 6552 acoustic features and was learned to predict the driver skill evaluation. As the figure shows, the distribution of the index of the high-skill group is higher than that of the low-skill group, confirming the possibility that driving skills can be estimated from these acoustic features.

In the future, if this research is further developed, with higher accuracy in predicting driving skills and the incidence of near-miss accidents in daily driving, it can be applied to shortening driving lessons for the elderly or as a tool for daily self-monitoring. Another possible application is to implement the system in automobiles to estimate the skills of the driver and provide assistance accordingly. Preventing accidents by elderly drivers is an essential social issue for the future aging of the

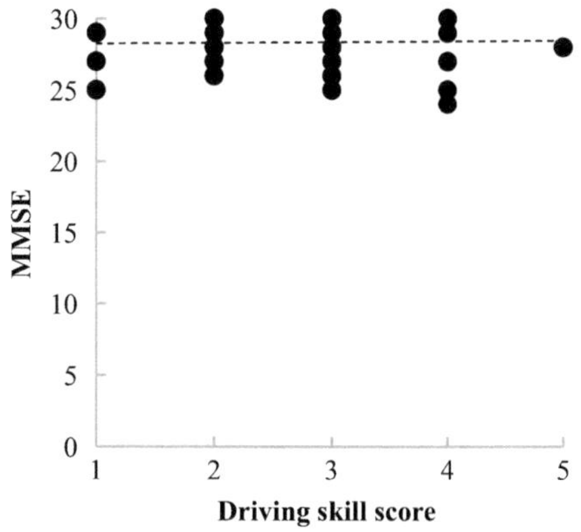

Fig. 20.3 Correlation between driving skill score and MMSE

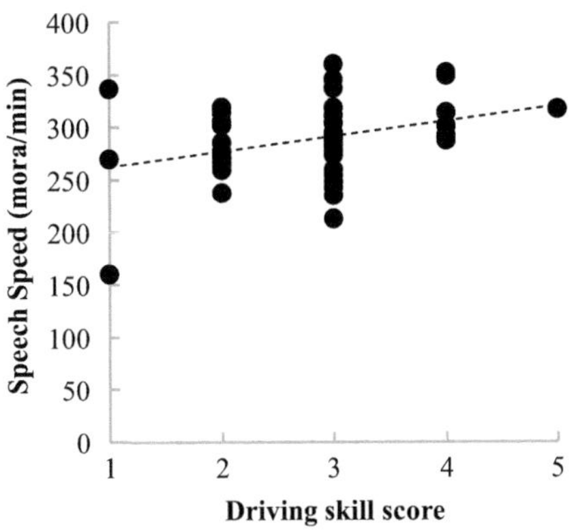

Fig. 20.4 Correlation between driving skill score and speech speed

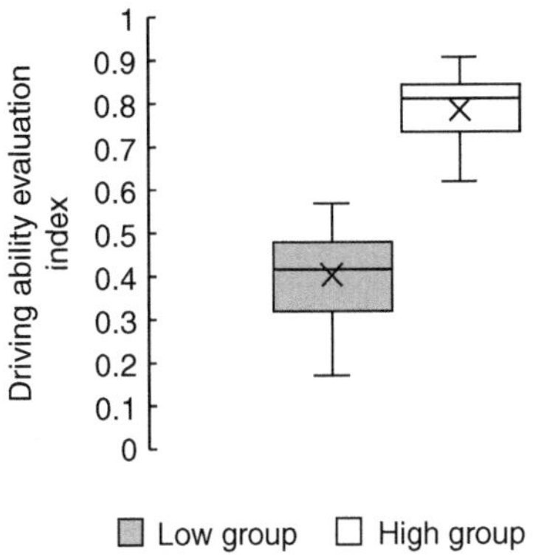

Fig. 20.5 Distribution of driving ability evaluation index by driving skills

world's population, and it is believed that this technology can solve this problem effectively.

20.4 Conclusion

In this chapter, two topics related to driving were introduced: first, the relationship between the mood and voice of the driver and, second, the driving skills of the driver and his or her voice. It is believed that both technologies can add new value to automobiles at a low cost. However, many problems remain to be studied, such as usage and how environmental noise affects the output. It is hoped that these studies will provide guidance for further research on applications.

References

Okazaki T (2016) Automotive application of verbal analysis [Japanese]. Mental Health 165:32–37. Japan Association for Mental Health
Tokuda K (2011) The validity of temporary mood scale [Japanese]. Ritsumeikan J Hum Sci 22(1):6

Chapter 21
COVID-19

Shinichi Tokuno

21.1 Introduction

The novel coronavirus infection (COVID-19) that originated in Wuhan, China, in December 2019 caused a worldwide pandemic. By December 2022, the cumulative number of infected people globally reached approximately 650 million, of which over 6.64 million lost their lives. With the unprecedented global spread of the disease, treatment initially focused on symptomatic treatment to save lives as effective drugs or vaccines had not yet been developed. To prevent infection during epidemics, countries enforced lockdowns and restricted individuals from leaving their homes in an attempt to reduce contact between people. These measures contributed to the isolation of individuals and caused economic stagnation, which, in turn, led to unemployment and reduced income, thus resulting in hardship and mental health problems. Since the beginning of the pandemic, various authorities, including the World health Organization (WHO), have been alerting the public of the need for mental health care (WHO 2020).

Moreover, the explosive increase in the number of infected people has strained medical and health resources in several countries, thus necessitating national triage. In numerous countries, people with mild illnesses are advised to be treated at home, and transportation to appropriate medical facilities is implemented according to the severity of the illness. Triage in disaster medical care is conducted in limited areas, and the determination of priority is based on medical examinations by physicians and others. However, if triage is to be conducted at the national level, diseases must be defined for accurate determination of severity, and remote determination is essential.

S. Tokuno (✉)
Department of Bioengineering, Graduate School of Engineering, The University of Tokyo, Bunkyo-ku, Tokyo, Japan
e-mail: tokuno@bioeng.t.u-tokyo.ac.jp

S. Tokuno, H. Nakamura (eds.), *Voice Biomarkers*,
https://doi.org/10.1007/978-981-96-3109-4_21

21.2 Mental Impact of Voluntary Restraint from Going Out

Three years after the COVID-19 pandemic, the mental impact of city lockdown on residents is being clarified (Guerfali and Zdanowicz 2022; Beharry 2022). However, although a mental impact was speculated at the beginning of the pandemic, the precise magnitude of this impact remains uncertain. Therefore, based on data obtained from a publicly available application (MNIMOSYS), we examined the extent to which Japanese people felt stressed by voluntary restrictions on going out (Omiya and Tokuno 2020). For more information on MIMOSYS, please refer to Chaps. 7, 8, 9, 10, 11, 12, and 13.

The analysis period was from January 1, 2020, to June 6, 2020. Of the 5246 users of the application, 126 who had been continuously analyzed automatically during their calls were included in the study. Of these, 8669 calls made by 90 people who obtained at least 3 call analyses during the analysis period were considered for the analysis in this study (Omiya and Tokuno 2020).

Figure 21.1 shows these results. Although short-term declines were observed in individual episodes associated with the pandemic, the decline associated with outing restrictions was significant.

Depressive tendencies were also observed.

In detail, as shown in Fig. 21.1, (i) the first case of infection was reported in Japan; (ii) Charter plane brings 206 Japanese back from Wuhan; (iii) the WHO declared a public health emergency, and the quarantine of the Diamond Princess cruise ship began; and (iv) elementary, middle, and high schools were closed and a

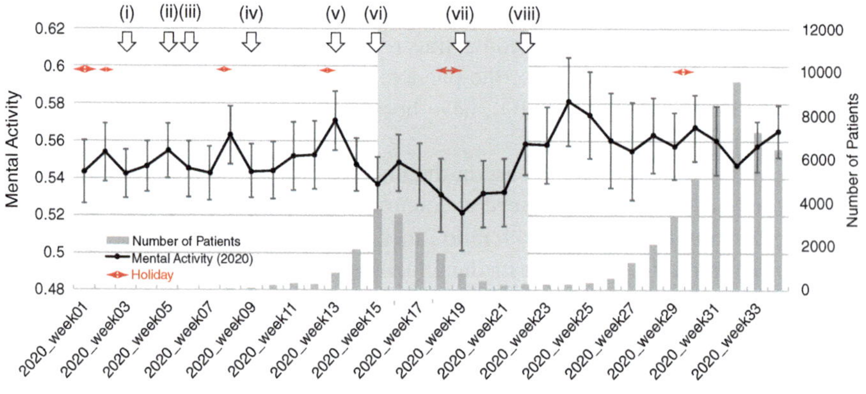

Fig. 21.1 COVID-19 pandemic changes in mental health indicators by voice. The graph shows weekly means and standard errors. The gray background represents the period of the outing restrictions. (i) First case of infection in Japan. (ii) A charter plane brought 206 Japanese people back from Wuhan. (iii) The WHO declared a public health emergency, and quarantine of the Diamond Princess cruise ship began. (iv) Elementary, middle, and high schools were closed. (v) The governor of Tokyo mentioned a lockdown. (vi) A state of emergency was declared (voluntary isolation at home). (vii) The state of emergency was extended. (viii) The state of emergency was lifted. No clear correlation was noted between the number of patients reported and mental activity. (Revised from Omiya and Tokuno 2020)

temporary decline in mental activity was observed; however, the fluctuation was not significant and the decline was transitory. Moreover, (v) the governor of Tokyo mentioned a lockdown and (vi) declared a state of emergency (voluntary isolation at home), which accelerated the decline. Subsequently, (vii) the state of emergency was extended; (viii) subsequently, it was lifted, thus leading to the recovery of mental activity to normal levels. Additionally, except for the period of self-restraint from outings, a transient increase in mental activity was observed immediately after the holidays. Thus, depressive tendencies were observed in situations in which there were direct restrictions on one's own life. No clear correlation was observed between the number of reported patients and mental activity.

In this country, no mandatory city lockdowns or restrictions on outings were implemented, and a month and a half of self-restraint on outings based on the people's initiative was implemented. Because people still reacted to depression, the impact on people with severe curfew restrictions, such as those implemented in some countries, was considerable.

21.3 Determination of COVID-19 Severity by Voice Biomarkers

With the increase in the number of infected patients, Japan has divided the severity of COVID-19 into four levels, as presented in Table 21.1, and defined moderate or higher disease as requiring treatment at a medical facility (MHLW 2023). Evidently from the table, blood oxygen saturation measured by a pulse oximeter is the most important and only objective indicator.

Table. 21.1 Classification of the severity of symptoms associated with COVID-19 infection

Severity	Oxygen saturation	Clinical state
Mild illness	$SpO_2 \geq 96\%$	No respiratory symptom (no findings consistent with pneumonia) or Cough only without any shortness of breath (no findings consistent with pneumonia)
Moderate illness I No respiratory failure	$93\% < SpO_2 < 96\%$	Shortness of breath and pneumonia findings
Moderate illness II Respiratory failure	$SpO_2 \leq 93\%$	Oxygen administration required
Acute		ICU admission or Ventilator needed

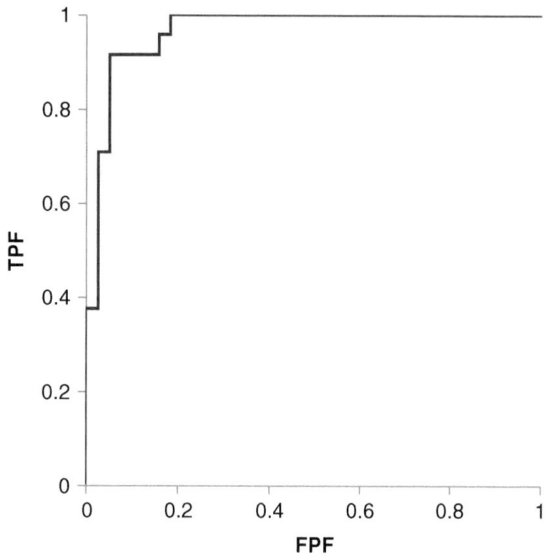

Fig. 21.2 COVID-19 severity determination by voice: ROC curve. AUC = 0.932, thus indicating extremely high discrimination accuracy. (Revised from Omiya et al. 2023)

However, with the increase in the number of infected patients, the distribution of pulse oximeters to all infected patients became challenging. Therefore, to develop a different and more convenient objective index, we attempted to determine the severity of COVID-19 using vocal biomarkers.

Patients aged 20 years or older with asymptomatic or mild infection with novel coronavirus who were treated at a care facility or home in Kanagawa Prefecture, Japan, from June 2021 to September 2022 were included. Patients whose symptoms worsened during treatment and who became moderately ill were also included. A study recruitment leaflet was distributed to the participants, and those interested in participating accessed the web through a QR code on the leaflet. Data were collected using a dedicated smartphone application to collect questionnaires on symptoms and other information along with voice recordings. A total of 659 participants were included in this study. Because the prevalent viral strains differed depending on the time of participation, the participants were matched for sex, age, and time of participation. Twenty-four patients with moderate disease and 38 patients with mild disease had valid voice and symptom recordings. The speech analysis was similar to the methods described in the previous chapters, with 13,998 speech features calculated using openSMILE and machine learning with LightGBM (Omiya et al. 2023); for more details, refer to Omiya's study.

As presented in Fig. 21.2 and Table 21.2, moderate and mild symptoms can be classified by voice with extremely high accuracy.

As this study targets language-independent sustained vowels as analysis phrases, it is independent of the native language. In addition, because this study does not analyze spontaneous speech, such as interviews or dialogues, it can be easily measured by a user without a measurer. Additionally, for medical personnel responsible

Table 21.2 COVID-19 severity determination by voice

		Predicted group	
		Mild illness	Moderate illness 1
Actual group	Mild illness	36	2
	Moderate illness 1	3	21

Sensitivity, 0.792; specificity, 0.947; accuracy, 0.887

for remote judgment, an increase in objective indicators is expected to facilitate judgment.

21.4 Summary

We demonstrated two uses of voice biomarkers in response to the COVID-19 pandemic: utilization in mental health and classification of disease severity.

Thus, voice biomarkers will be an effective tool in telemedicine.

References

Beharry M (2022) Pediatric anxiety and depression in the time of COVID-19. Pediatr Ann 51(4):e154–e160. https://doi.org/10.3928/19382359-20220317-01

Guerfali Y, Zdanowicz N (2022) Depression during COVID-19 pandemic: is there an emergency? Psychiatr Danub 34(Suppl 8):14–17

Ministry of Health, Labor and Welfare, Japan (2023) A guide to medical care of COVID-19, Version 9.0. [Cited 8 August 2023]. Available online: https://www.mhlw.go.jp/content/000936655.pdf (Japanese)

Omiya Y, Tokuno S (2020) How much of an impact did COVID-19 self-isolation measures have on mental health? Asian J Psychiatr 54:102445. https://doi.org/10.1016/j.ajp.2020.102445

Omiya Y, Mizuguchi D, Tokuno S (2023) Distinguish the severity of illness associated with novel coronavirus (COVID-19) infection via sustained vowel speech features. Int J Environ Res Public Health 20(4):3415. https://doi.org/10.3390/ijerph20043415

World Health Organization (2020) Mental health and psychosocial considerations during the COVID-19 Outbreak [Cited 8 August 2023]. Available online: https://www.who.int/docs/default-source/coronaviruse/mental-health-considerations.pdf?sfvrsn=6d3578af_2

GPSR Compliance

The European Union's (EU) General Product Safety Regulation (GPSR) is a set of rules that requires consumer products to be safe and our obligations to ensure this.

If you have any concerns about our products, you can contact us on ProductSafety@springernature.com

In case Publisher is established outside the EU, the EU authorized representative is:

Springer Nature Customer Service Center GmbH
Europaplatz 3
69115 Heidelberg, Germany

Batch number: 10726135

Printed by Printforce, the Netherlands